The Fat Flush Cookbook

ANN LOUISE GITTLEMAN
Ph.D., C.N.S.

McGraw-Hill

New York / Chicago / San Francisco / Lisbon / London
Madrid / Mexico City / Milan / New Delhi / San Juan
Seoul / Singapore / Sydney / Toronto

ISBN 0-07-140794-4 (HC)   18 19 20   DOC/DOC   0 9 8 7
ISBN 0-07-143367-8 (PB)   6 7 8 9 0   DOC/DOC   0 9 8 7

McGraw-Hill books are available at special discounts to use as premiums and sales promotions, or for use in corporate training programs. For more information, please write to the Director of Special Sales, Professional Publishing, McGraw-Hill, Two Penn Plaza, New York, NY 10121-2298. Or contact your local bookstore.

This book is for educational purposes. It is not intended as a substittute for medical advice. Please consult a qualified health care professional for individual health and medical advice. Neither McGraw-Hill nor the author shall have any responsibility for any adverse effects arising directly or indirectly as a result of the information provided in this book.

Throughout this book, trademarked names are used. Rather than put a trademark symbol after every occurrence of a trademarked name, we use names in an editorial fashion only and to the benefit of the trademark owner, with no intention of infringement of the trademark. Where such designations appear in this book, they have been printed with initial capitals.

 This book is printed on recycled, acid-free paper containing a minimum of 50% recycled de-inked paper.

Library of Congress Cataloging-in-Publication Data

Gittleman, Ann Louise.
  The fat flush cookbook / Ann Louise Gittleman.
    p. cm.
Includes index.
  ISBN 0-07-140794-4 (hardcover : alk. paper)
  1. Reducing diets—Recipes.   I. Title.
  RM222.2 .G5372 2003
  613.2'5—dc21   2002013398

Contents

Acknowledgments

Fat Flush has brought me many blessings and in many respects has represented a turning point in my life—both professionally and personally.

I am grateful that the writing of the first book *The Fat Flush Plan* in the spring and summer of 2001 enabled me to spend some time in my hometown of West Hartford, Connecticut, where I had the opportunity to visit and say good-bye (although I didn't know it would be a final farewell) to two of my dearest uncles, George Berkowitz and Jacob Kriwitsky. Shortly thereafter, my uncle Ben Kritwitsky also passed away, so this time in my life has been a crossroads on many levels.

Last summer was also the last time I saw my long-time literary agent, Mike Cohn, who passed away in February of 2002. *The Fat Flush Plan* was dedicated to Mike, who, in great measure, was responsible for my writing career. When I asked his widow Suzanne how Mike really felt about the dedication, she told me that "if he read it once a day, he read it ten times out loud." I will miss Mike's wisdom, direction, and unerring support of my work—not to mention those early 6 a.m. telephone calls when he had good news to report.

My deepest thanks and gratitude to the entire McGraw-Hill team for making this cookbook and the Fat Flush phenomenon a reality. My McGraw-Hill dream team includes my talented editor Nancy Hancock, whose commitment to my work and creative guidance is unsurpassed. She was right. And from the bottom of my heart I would like to acknowledge my publisher, Philip Ruppel; the director of marketing, Lynda Luppino; the marketing manager, Eileen Lamadore; publicity manager, Ann Pryor; subsidiary rights director, Irina Lumelsky; international sales and marketing director, Chitra Bopardikar; translation rights, Allyson Arias; special sales, Linda Babat; editing supervisor, Scott Kurtz; McGraw-Hill/Ryerson publicist, Doug Blair; and Alan Sears, the McGraw-Hill rep for the Pacific Northwest. I hope you will all remain part of my newfound literary family for a very long time.

I wish to express my enduring thanks to all of my supporters on the home front headed up by Stuart K. Gittleman, the business arm of First Lady of Nutrition, Inc. Stuart, as many of you know who email, call, or write me is simply *the best* regarding follow-up, follow-through, and professionalism. He is kind and considerate, and a consummate pro. I should know. I am also his sister

I must thank Lan Hahn and Debbie Nelson-Judd here in the Northwest for coming onto the Fat Flush scene at the right time. Also, my deepest appreciation to journalist Susan Hamilton for her great Fat Flush coverage in *Northwest Woman* and *The Inlander*. Kudos to Joe and Sara Hamilton of Pilgrim Health Foods in Spokane for conducting bimonthly Fat Flush classes to support the community under my supervision. And to those of you in all the other locales around the country and around the globe who are spreading the Fat Flush message through special events, classes, and Fat Flush dinners—thank you.

Heartfelt thanks to my faithful Fat Flush community leaders. My sincere thanks to the remarkable ladies who have worked both the ivillage Fat Flush board and the Forum 7 days a week, 24 hours a day—especially Jackie Scott, Mary Dodge, Kathy Jensen, Barbara Anderson, Linda Leekley, Carol Ackerman, and Linda Shapiro.

Rose Grandy, Kari Wheaton, Jackie Scott, and Linda Shapiro provided very helpful assistance with the recipe selection, development, test tasting, and review of these recipes so I know that other Fat Flushers like them will find the recipes doable, usable, as well as fairly quick and easy. Kari's creativity and cooking expertise contributed in no small measure to the entrée section.Thanks also to Ellen Buier for her culinary contributions and generosity; to Claudia Krevat for her recipe contributions; to Pete Tobin, culinary instructor; and to Edith Gittleman for her vast cooking talents and attention to detail regarding clarity of cooking instructions.

My significant other, the cowboy from Texas , deserves a medal for putting up with crazy writing schedules and creative chaos. Just remember Sir James—forever is as far as I'll go.

Thank you also to my dear Fat Flush followers. You have turned out in record numbers at book signings, lectures, and demonstrations to show your support. Many of you have been with me since the very beginning, back in 1988 when *Beyond Pritikin* hit the stands. You have followed my career through all of my books and have the tattered, torn pages to prove it!

And to my dear friends who have been there with me through all the challenging times and have rejoiced with me during the triumphs: Liz and Monroe Paul and Herb, Dianna, and Dick; Diane and Roy; Lena and John; Helen and Bill; Linda and Malcolm; Ann, Signe, and Gillian. These extraordinary people epitomize this definition: "A friend is someone who knows the song in your heart and sings it back to you when you have forgotten how it goes."

Introduction

As everyone who is familiar with *The Fat Flush Plan* knows, I am totally committed to helping people cleanse and purify their systems and get trim, fit, and healthy. Since launching *The Fat Flush Plan* in 2001, I've learned so much about the real life applications of Fat Flush and how it is changing people's lives that a companion cookbook seemed like the natural and logical next step. *The Fat Flush Plan* details my weight loss/lifestyle system that evolved over 15 years from my own personal experience, the success of my clients, and the science behind the five hidden weight gain factors that sabotage weight loss. This cookbook will help you translate and put together the unique dietary components of the system into real life breakfast, lunch, dinner, and snacks. And while I believe that it's what's inside a person's heart and soul that really counts, this doesn't change the reality that your weight affects your health and that your physical appearance affects how you feel and the way you feel about yourself.

In fact, based upon the latest government statistics on overweight and obesity, a Fat Flush Plan cookbook is quite timely, indeed. Nearly 130 million people or 61 percent of all Americans now weigh too much. Over half the adult population in the United States is overweight with nearly a third classified as obese. Too much weight, plain and simple, is directly connected to heart disease, diabetes, and arthritis.

But in these days after September 11, Americans seem to be paying more attention to comfort and feel-good foods (think lasagna and sweets) rich in calories, undesirable fats, and sugars rather than the foods that provide the vital nutrients we need to maintain a healthy weight and protect overall health. So my challenge as a nutritionist in developing the *Fat Flush Plan Cookbook* was not only to help you lose or control weight with the Fat Flush principles and concepts, but also, at the same time, to treat you to home cooked, absolutely satisfying meals with recipes that are comforting, cozy, and healthy without your feeling deprived.

In addition, there is another major aspect to consider—time, or the lack of it. On a daily basis I receive hundreds of faxes, emails, and Internet postings from readers from all walks of life with one common denominator—they are all racing against the clock. Many of them have full-time jobs that are sometimes 24/7, they are working strange shifts, they commute to work, they try to keep workout appointments at the gym, they are raising a family, and they still want to reward themselves with fast, easy, great-tasting recipes that won't pack on the pounds.

So when you said you wanted more Fat Flush recipes that were appropriate for each of the three phases of the plan (but most especially ones that could be used for the more stringent phase 1) and that were speedy without sacrificing taste or quality, I listened. And the result is a three-diets-in-one cookbook containing an unbeatable collection of weight loss recipes which, for the most part, take less than half an hour to prepare yet are wonderfully aromatic and full of flavor because of the tantalizing and unusual use of herbs and spices on the food itself or in dressings, pâtés, marinades, and condiments.

Not only will you flush away fat and drop a dress (or pants) size or two in the process, but the *Fat Flush Plan Cookbook* is guaranteed to open up a whole new world of eating, cooking, and exotic flavorings that are good for weight loss and overall well-being. Whether its a main dish like Tangy Chicken with Tomatillos or a condiment such as Cran-Jewel Ketchup, a dessert like Vanilla Peaches or a topping such as Minty Dill Pesto, the breakfasts, entrees, soups, side dishes, dressings, beverages, condiments, and sweet indulgences within these pages will spice up your life and enhance your health.

Did you know that the average spice rack in an American kitchen contains around 15 different types of herbs and spices? So you don't have to look any farther than your own kitchen to add pizzazz to your recipes and find proven metabolism boosters and fat burners (cayenne, ginger, garlic, mustard, cinnamon) to wake everything up. Not everybody in the country has an herb garden or can locate fresh herbs in the grocery store, so, with the exception of the more easily available fresh ginger, parsley, and cilantro, most of the recipes call for the more convenient and potent dried versions that most likely are already in your kitchen cupboard. (True herb lovers are always welcome to use fresh, of course. It takes 1 tablespoon of the fresh herb or spice to equal 1 teaspoon of the dried, crushed herb. Fresh is usually three times as potent as the dried version.)

I promise that the *Fat Flush Plan Cookbook* will make it easier than ever for you to meet your weight loss goals despite your hectic lifestyle. And you will be able to do this without sugar, salt, and undesirable fats. So what are you waiting for? It's time to revisit and rediscover what the Fat Flush phenomenon is all about, how the choices have evolved, which herbs and spices are the best for weight loss and healing, and how to Fat Flush your kitchen for those fast and fabulous recipes that are just pages away.

1 The Fat Flush Phenomenon

As hundreds of thousands of satisfied Fat Flushers already know, the Fat Flush concepts represent a paradigm shift in weight loss and lasting weight control by targeting the liver as your number 1 weight loss roadblock. In fact, believe it or not, nothing you do to control your weight is as important as keeping your liver healthy.

This is the biggest weight loss story in years. And that's why I believe that *The Fat Flush Plan* became a *New York Times* and *USA Today* bestseller within the first two months of publication. It's also the reason that the Fat Flush interactive messaging board has become so busy on iVillage.com, the top destination for women online, and has received up to 700,000 unique visitors per month.

To further assist you in your Fat Flush journey, I have created this companion cookbook with easy and zesty recipes that are designed to increase metabolism, flush out bloat, and speed up or maintain fat loss. And that's not all you will achieve. The Fat Flush principles and ingredients incorporated in these recipes extend beyond just weight loss. The added bonus of internal cleansing, liver detoxification, and body purification will provide you with unexpected mental and emotional benefits such as mental alertness, increased energy, appetite control, satiety without food cravings, and a noticeable decrease in depression, irritability, and anxiety.

There are 200 unique Fat Flush recipes and snacks—many of them ready in less than 20 minutes—which are easily identified for each of the three weight loss phases of the Plan. For example, the phase 1: Two-Week Fat Flush recipes are designed for accelerated weight loss; the phase 2: Ongoing Fat Flush recipes are designed for transitional weight loss wherein more food choices are provided; while phase 3: Lifestyle Eating recipes are designed for a lifetime plan to help you stay fit permanently without having to give up your favorite foods.

Keep in mind that the entrées, soups, salads, dressings, condiments, beverages, and even sweet indulgences contain the world's best fat flushing ingredients (such as, cranberries, flaxseed oil, apple cider vinegar, and lemons) plus cleansing and metabolism-boosting herbs and spices (such as ginger, cayenne, mustard, cinnamon, cloves, bay leaves, and fennel), which are far more than just flavor enhancers.

Every day science reveals how some of the original Fat Flush staples and spices, such as cranberries, apple cider vinegar, ginger, and cilantro, are not only good for weight loss but also provide spectacular health benefits as well. Just before *The Fat Flush Plan* was released at the end of 2001, a highly publicized study appeared in the *Journal of Agricultural and Food Chemistry*, which ranked cranberries as one of the most healthful foods to consume. Scientists at the University of Scranton proclaimed that cranberries, when compared to 19 other fruits commonly eaten in the United States, have extraordinarily high amounts of a certain antioxidant called phenols, which protect against heart disease, cancer, and stroke.

Apple cider vinegar—long heralded in folk medicine for its cleansing and therapeutic effects on obesity and arthritis because of its high concentration of potassium, trace minerals, and enzymes—has been the subject of university studies and has been found to live up to its legend. A recent Arizona State University trial found that participants who consumed as little as 1 1/2 tablespoons of the vinegar ate 200 fewer calories at the following meal.

Ginger, a primary fat flushing herb that boosts metabolism and reduces fatty buildup, has recently been found by Danish scientists to head off migraines and ease arthritic aches and pains.

Another Fat Flush favorite, cilantro, also known as Mexican parsley, is more than just a frequent flavor enhancer in the recipes. It has been found to help with the removal of heavy metals from the system, primarily mercury, which can negatively affect the central nervous system.

The Fat Flush recipes have been specifically created with many of these superstar health foods and spices as well as lots of colorful veggies, fruits, lean proteins, and satisfying oils to zap *all* the five hidden weight gain stumbling blocks, which underlie the excess poundage currently plaguing over 114 million Americans.

My research, online counseling, and hands-on experience with nearly 10 million dieters over the past 20 years have revealed that the real culprits behind weight gain are not simply a lack of will power, overeating, or underexercising as you have been told. They are far more insidious and alarming.

Here's a thumbnail sketch of the *five hidden weight gain factors* which provide the scientific foundation behind the Fat Flush philosophy:

1. **Your tired, toxic liver.** The number 1 weight loss stumbling block, a liver overloaded with pollutants and toxins, cannot efficiently burn body fat, and thus it will sabotage your weight loss efforts. The recipes eliminate all liver damaging elements. They omit caffeine, sugar, trans fats (hydrogenated and partially hydrogenated vegetable fats and oils) from fried foods, margarine, vegetable shortenings and commercial vegetable oils, and yeast-based foods (soy sauce and most vine-

gars). And they feature liver-loving ingredients like cruciferous vegetables (broccoli, Brussels sprouts, and kale), eggs (high in amino acids which are needed for the liver to break down fats), and liver-supporting herbs and spices such as garlic, onion, and ginger root.

2. **When fat is not fat.** The number 2 weight loss stumbling block—waterlogged tissues—results when you consume too little water and protein and from food sensitivities, hormonal fluctuations, and certain medications. You'll find that filtered water is a major component in all the diet phase protocols because of its purifying properties and ability to remove wastes from the body. Powerful (yet so simple and easy to make) protein-based recipes are provided with beef, chicken, fish, eggs, tofu, and whey. The latest health food darling—ruby red cranberries—plays a feature role in many of the condiments, such as Cranberry-Catsup, and the dishes, such as Cran-Raspberry Sauce. In addition, the majority of the recipes eliminate two of the food groups that can promote water retention—gluten-rich grains and dairy products. The flaxseed oil featured in the salad dressings acts as a natural hormone balancer and as replacement therapy. Parsley, cilantro, fennel, and anise are sprinkled throughout the recipes because of their diuretic qualities.

3. **The fear of eating fat.** The number 3 weight loss stumbling block—lack of fat-burning fats—flies in the face of everything you have been told for the past 20 years. The truth is that certain fats [like flaxseed oil, gamma linoleic acid (GLA) from evening primrose oil, borage or black currant seed oil, and conjugated linoleic acid (CLA)] can accelerate fat burning, trigger fat loss, and provide long-term satiety while maintaining lean muscle mass. While the GLA and CLA fats are taken as dietary supplements, nutty ground up flaxseeds (in addition to the flaxseed oil that serves as a basis for delightfully light dressings and vinaigrettes) are contained in many of the breakfast smoothie recipes and their variations. I also encourage you to select meats from grass-fed cattle whenever possible. This is the best natural food source of CLA.

4. **Excess insulin and excess inflammation.** The number 4 weight loss stumbling block—excess insulin and excess inflammation—are fat-promoting hormones created by foods high in carbohydrates. The Fat Flush program combats excess insulin and excess inflammation by providing a diet equation of 40 percent total calories from anti-inflammatory essential (and blood sugar stabilizing) fats, with the rest of calories divided between powerful protein dishes (which produce the hormone glucagons that counteract insulin) and low glycemic (or slow-acting) carbs from rainbow colored veggies and fruits, Mother Nature's anti-inflammatory foods. The Fat Flush dietary approach increases insulin efficiency and transforms the body into a fat-burning, not fat-building, mode.

5. **Stress as fat maker.** The number 5 weight loss stumbling block—stress—functions as a fat maker because the stress hormone cortisol, like insulin, is a major fat-promoting hormone. Cortisol, however, has a propensity for stimulating central fat or tummy fat. Fat Flush recipes feature lightning fast meals and quick and easy snacks that can correct the stress fat cycle by reducing cortisol levels through proper meal timing. The key here is to eat something about every three hours *before* you are hungry. The meals-in-minutes techniques help to balance blood sugar throughout the day, thereby avoiding cravings and fat storage.

COUNTDOWN TO FAT FLUSH

You're getting closer and closer to the next level of the Fat Flush experience. The next chapter includes comprehensive food options for each level of the plan with recommended portions to help you make the program more convenient and more practical than ever. Then I'll help you set up your Fat Flush kitchen with some suggestions on the best time-saving utensils and equipment to have on hand to maximize your results. And, before your know it, you'll be ready to start on that fast and fabulous food. Just make sure you also make some time for shopping—clothes shopping, that is, because you'll soon be ready for a fabulous new wardrobe!

2 The Fat Flush Plan Evolves

Fat Flush is really an eating evolution.

As many of you already know, a foundational and comprehensive list of acceptable foods, beverages, spices, and brand names for each of the three phases of the program is provided in *The Fat Flush Plan*. Also provided are sample menu plans and culinary ideas for each phase. As new research becomes available, there will be new herbs, spices, foods, sweeteners, and brand names that I will be adding periodically to your Fat Flush repertoire. Many of you will be delighted to note that in developing the recipes for this book, I have introduced additional Fat-Flush–friendly foods and seasoning options (and in some cases additional brand names) that are in line with the plan's cleansing, weight loss, and lifestyle principles. You'll also find a list of new ingredients for Phase 3 and special-occasion cooking.

And so, what else is new?

BEFORE YOU BEGIN, OR IF YOU HAVE FALLEN OFF THE FAT FLUSH WAGON

During the week before you begin phase 1 for the first time or before you start phase 1 all over again, there are many practical ways to prepare your body for the Fat Flush experience. As I explain in *The Fat Flush Plan*, tapering off alcohol, coffee, tea, colas, and other soft drinks (which are major liver stressors) and substituting herbal coffees is probably the single most important thing you can do to prepare your system for cleansing. This step will also help to forestall the withdrawal symptoms of fatigue, headaches, irritability, and increased hunger once you are on the full-fledged program.

Besides getting caffeine out of your life, I have learned that the next two next biggest Fat Flush challenges are getting rid of sugar and getting the salt out. So, let's take out the sugar first!

In the chapter entitled "Five Hidden Weight Gain Factors" in *The Fat Flush Plan*, you learned that white sugar (and white flour and white rice which are metabolized like sugar) adversely affect your blood sugar and insulin levels as well as trigger yeast overgrowth. While high blood sugar, excess insulin, and excess yeast can lead to a slew of health challenges like adult-onset diabetes, cardiovascular disease, and impaired immunity, they can also sabotage your weight loss efforts.

Whether you are trying to lose weight or improve your overall health, here's what you need to do to get started so your transition to the phase 1: Two-Week Fat Flush will be as pleasant as possible

PRE FAT FLUSH: ELEVEN TRANSITIONAL TIPS TO GET THE SUGAR OUT

If you are hooked on sugar, these tips are absolutely essential for your Fat Flush success:

1. *Right now,* stop adding sugar to foods such as cereal and fruits and to any of your drinks—even those herbal coffee substitutes or herbal teas you are now using. All forms of sugar, sugar alcohols, and artificial sweeteners are out for this transitional phase. The noncaloric sugar alcohols (such as mannitol, sorbitol, and xylitol) found in sugar-free chewing gums are often the cause of cramps, diarrhea, and bloating. Artificial sweeteners like Aspartame (also known as Equal or NutraSweet) can increase both sugar and carbohydrate cravings by blocking production of serotonin. Insufficient serotonin creates more sugar and carbohydrate cravings, which can then increase the likelihood of binging. Watch out for all the fancy names for any of the above, like dehydrated cane crystals, cane juice crystals, cane sugar, caramel, corn syrup, corn syrup solids, dextrose, diastase, fructose, fruit juice and fruit juice concentrates, invert sugar, lactose, malt syrup, maltodextrin, maltose, sorghum syrup, regular sugar, raw sugar, turbinado sugar, and brown sugar. (Ideally, these should not be consumed at all, unless they are listed right near the end of the ingredients—ideally way after the first five ingredients.)

2. Get rid of processed carbohydrates from your kitchen starting today. As I mention previously but this is well worth repeating, refined carbohydrates in the form of white rice, white bread, and white pasta (the "wicked whites") are rapidly converted to sugars in the body and upset the body's blood sugar and fat-controlling systems. Keeping these products out of the house is a very simple yet most effective way to maintain a well-balanced blood sugar level for long-term energy and the avoidance of hunger (and temptations).

3. Foodwise, just remember to go with unrefined and unprocessed as much as possible. This is the *only* way to ensure that you are really reducing your sugar intake, especially the hidden sugars in sauces, cereals, dressings, and such. Most vegetables and fruits as well as chicken, meat, fish, tofu, and eggs are as sugar free as you can get. The

naturally occurring sugars present in legumes, grains, vegetables, fruits, nuts, and seeds are combined with fiber and other nutrients which help to balance your blood sugar by slowing down the body's absorption and assimilation of the natural sugars present.

4. Dilute even the natural sweeteners or naturally sweetened foods whenever you can. If you are a health nut already and are using healthful sweeteners like barley malt or brown rice syrup, for example, then dilute these concentrated sweeteners with water.

5. Avoid any food with the label "fat free," the marketing trick that makes you think such foods may help you lose weight but have actually contributed to our increasing weight and health problems. (Remember that section in *The Fat Flush Plan* in the "Five Hidden Weight Gain Factors" chapter that discusses the consequences of the fear of eating fat, even the right—fat burning fats?) When "fat free" is on the label, you can be sure to find lots of sugar in various disguises ending with "-ose" like sucrose, glucose, dextrose, and levulose to improve the taste factor. Excess amounts of sugar that are not balanced with protein and fat cause the pancreas to release insulin, the body's main fat storage hormone.

6. The more natural, the better the food for you. So, load up on fresh veggies and fruits. The more processed a food may be (think potato chips and even orange juice), the more it will tend to raise your blood sugar because the fiber and nutrients are missing.

7. Make a vow to ingest foods *only* with 0 to 4 grams of sugars per serving. Become a sugar sleuth. To cut the sugar out, you have to know where it is hiding first. There's no way around it. If you are still buying packaged foods, you have to pay attention to what's in them. Three quarters of the sugars Americans ingest are "hidden" in processed foods, so you have to become a health detective. Learn to read those labels and search for the various names for sugar itemized in number 1 above.

8. Now that we are on the topic of labels, note that the label "sugar free" means that the food contains fewer than 0.5 grams of sugar. The labels "no added sugar," "without added sugar," and "no sugar added" mean that no sugar or ingredients containing sugars were added during the processing or packing of the products and that the product has no ingredients that were made with added sugars, such as jams, jellies, or concentrated fruit juices. The term "reduced sugar" means that the product contains at least 25 percent less sugar than the original product.

9. Start eating for taste and good health. The human body requires only about 2 teaspoons of sugar in the bloodstream at any one time. You can easily meet this requirement with fresh fruits and veggies, protein, and fat.

10. Listen to your body. Think about what happens when you eat that decadently chocolaty dessert. You may feel an initial high, but an hour later the irritability, depression, and lethargy set in; what is your body telling you? Try to choose foods that make you feel good for the long term—mentally, emotionally, and physically.

11. Start to eat regular, balanced meals and minisnacks. Think protein (eggs, poultry, beef, fish, lamb, tofu), veggies (the more vibrant the color, the better), and quality fats (flaxseed and olive oil) at every meal. Concentrate on fresh fruits twice a day between meals.

PREFAT FLUSH: TEN TRANSITIONAL TIPS TO GET THE SALT OUT

Sugar is on its way out of your diet once again. Now, if you are still addicted to salt, listen up. As you already know, excess salt is a primary dietary culprit for waterlogged tissues—one of the five hidden weight gain factors discussed in *The Fat Flush Plan*. Excessive consumption of salt is also linked to strokes, hypertension, and a variety of cardiovascular problems.

The following transitional tips suggest simple ways to shake the salt so that once you begin your Fat Flush journey, you will not be missing it:

1. During the week before you begin Fat Flush, reduce the amount of salt you use in cooking. The salt added in cooking accounts for more than 40 percent of the sodium we consume. Try to reduce the salt called for in recipes by at least one-quarter to one-half until by the end of the week you are using no salt in cooking at all.

2. Add salt to foods *after* cooking for heightened flavor and less sodium. Did you know that salt added before or during cooking doesn't taste as salty as salt that is added after cooking? Why? The salty flavor rapidly dissipates in the cooking process.

3. There are 2000 milligrams of sodium in a teaspoon of salt. This amount is more than sufficient for the majority of Americans in a single day.

4. Become a salt sleuth. Like sugar, the overwhelming majority of the salt we consume is cleverly "hidden" in processed and refined foods. Salt can be disguised in lots of ways: sodium alginate, sodium aluminum sulfate, sodium ascorbate, sodium benzoate, sodium bisulfite, sodium carboxymethyl cellulose, sodium caseinate, sodium nitrite, sodium propionate, sodium saccharin, baking powder, baking soda, disodium phosphate, and monosodium glutamate (MSG).

5. Focus on buying foods that carry the label "sodium free" or "low sodium." The sodium-free foods contain 35 or fewer milligrams of sodium per serving. The low-sodium foods contain 140 milligrams per serving.

6. According to Asian medicine, salt cravings can signal your body's attempt to balance excessive sugar or alcohol in the diet. Since you will be eliminating both sugar and alcohol in this pre Fat Flush transitional phase, your salt cravings should disappear gradually.

7. If you still find yourself craving salt even though you have cut out both sugar and alcohol, then this may be a sign of burned out adrenal glands (your stress glands). You can strengthen these glands by eating frequent minimeals, learning relaxation techniques, and for those of you who have been diagnosed with low blood pressure, a pinch of salt can be helpful.

8. Get used to garlic, cayenne, ginger, mustard, cinnamon, cloves, and dill as tasty replacements for regular table salt. These healthful herbs and spices can heighten food flavors naturally as well as aid your weight loss efforts by revving up metabolism and helping to balance blood sugar.

9. Focus on the K factor. The symbol "K" stands for potassium, the mineral that counteracts excess sodium in the diet. Potassium is found in all Fat Flush veggies and fruits—especially tomatoes, squash, and citrus fruits.

10. Kick the salt habit by *overstimulating* other tastes. Use cider vinegar and the juices of lemons and limes liberally on your salads, in your veggies, and in marinades.

Now that you know the secrets of how to get both sugar and salt out of your diet for the pre Fat Flush phase, there's even better news about what you can look forward to on the Fat Flush Plan.

INCLUDE CRAN IN YOUR PLAN

You will find that cranberries themselves—in addition to cran-water and unsweetened cranberry juice—are now part of the program in every phase. These ruby-red jewels are chock full of important antioxidants. In light of the new research that has been published by researchers at the University of Scranton, I have created new and delicious recipes in which they play an intriguing role.

ALL PHASES: POMEGRANATE AND POMEGRANATE JUICE ALTERNATIVE

Another added fat flushing food in the Fat Flush Evolution is the pomegranate. One-half of a pomegranate or 1 small pomegranate is now a new fruit exchange on all phases of the program! The word *pomegranate* is translated as "apple with many seeds" from the ancient Hebrew. This delectable and exotic fruit may actually date back to the Garden of Eden. Scholars now believe that Eve's apple was actually a pomegranate.

Not only is this exotic fruit steeped in religious significance, mythology, and legend (the pomegranate was said to be the favorite food of the gods and symbolized long life, regeneration, and marriage), but it has some modern-day scientific backing that is very impressive. Clinical studies have shown that pomegranate juice, similar in some respects to cranberry juice, has demonstrated incredibly high antioxidant activity. In fact, only 4 ounces of unsweetened pomegranate juice per day can help reduce and may even reverse arterial lesions. Three published studies in highly reputable journals (*The Journal of Nutrition*, August 2001; *Atherosclerosis*, 2001; and *The American Journal of Clinical Nutrition*, May 2000) revealed the amazingly positive impact of pomegranate juice intake on cardiovascular health.

Notwithstanding the Garden of Eden connection, of course, the science is the real reason I have added both the pomegranate and unsweetened pomegranate juice to the Fat Flush protocols—with this caveat: While the pomegranate itself can be used as a fruit exchange for everybody for all phases, the unsweetened pomegranate juice should be only used for those who are allergic to cranberry or who live outside of the United States, where cranberry is simply unavailable. I cannot vouch for the fat-burning benefits of pomegranate juice, unlike the unsweetened cranberry juice with which I have had nearly ten years of clinical experience.

So, having said that, let's say that you are allergic to cranberries and will be using the pomegranate juice. If you are on phase 1, The Two Week Fat Flush, you can use 2 ounces of unsweetened pomegranate juice (available in supermarkets and health food stores) as an alternative for the 4 ounces of straight cranberry juice used to make up your cran-water. (By the way, it is not as tangy as the unsweetened cranberry—therefore it does not need any sweetener at all, not even Stevia Plus.)

HERE'S HOW TO USE THE UNSWEETENED POMEGRANATE JUICE FOR THOSE ALLERGIC TO CRANBERRIES

Instead of 28 ounces of plain water and 4 ounces of unsweetened cranberry juice, you will be making up a blend of 30 ounces of plain water and 2 ounces of unsweetened pomegranate juice for each of your two bottles.

For the Long Life Cocktail in phases 2 and 3, you may choose to use 2 ounces of the unsweetened pomegranate juice as an alternative for the 4 ounces of unsweetened cranberry juice and to use 6 ounces of water rather than the 4 ounces of water called for with the unsweetened cranberry juice.

Here's an easy cran water to pom water conversion table:

CRAN WATER	POM WATER
4 ounces unsweetened cranberry juice	2 ounces unsweetened pom juice
28 ounces plain water for 2 bottles	30 ounces (2 bottles) plain water

ALL PHASES: NEW SPICE AND VEGGIES

Do note that turmeric, that bright yellow spice that gives color and zip to curries and is also a powerful liver protector packed with antioxidants, is A-OK for every phase of Fat Flush cooking. And guess what? You will also find more veggies selections represented in the cookbook too. You may now have unlimited (unless otherwise noted) raw or steamed artichoke (1 whole or 4 artichoke hearts), rhubarb (1 cup), hearts of palm, tomatillos, snow peas, and jalapeños (a mildly hot green chile pepper), including one that may not be familiar to you—burdock. In Chinese medicine, burdock, a medicinal root vegetable, is known for its purifying and, blood cleansing properties. It also stimulates the secretion of bile and is very helpful for diabetics because it contains inulin, a sweet tasting soluble fiber that has blood sugar regulating and laxative benefits. (It is featured in a recipe called Carrot Burdock Stir Sauté on page 137.)

CREAM OF TARTAR

Another ingredient that has been added to the protocol for All Phases is cream of tartar (potassium bitartrate)—the meringue and soufflé stabilizer. (It helps to keep beaten egg whites foamy.) A by-product of wine making, cream of tartar is an old-time remedy for cleansing the blood stream and aiding regularity (it can be found in laxatives). So, the mildly acidic cream of tartar has many practical and therapeutic benefits for Fat Flush.

THE FAT FLUSH FLAX FACTOR—FIBER IT UP!

I think you will be very pleased to see the expanded culinary usage of flaxseeds in the ground and milled forms. If you are currently using the ground or milled flaxseed as your fiber component in the Long Life Cocktail, you now have the option to use your recommended dosage of 2 tablespoons (total) per day in food preparation. For example, there are recipes that use toasted ground or milled flaxseeds as coatings, toppings, and garnishes. For a change of pace, you are welcome to get creative and use the flaxseed component of these recipes to fulfill the daily Long Life Cocktail fiber allotment or your flaxseed oil requirement (it takes 3 tablespoons of the ground seed to equal 1 tablespoon of the oil) for the partial amount or total recommended amount.

As you already know from *The Fat Flush Plan*, the benefits of flaxseed are remarkable. Besides being high in the metabolism stoking, fat-burning Omega-3s, flaxseeds are a rich source of both soluble and insoluble fiber. The soluble fiber helps in stabilizing blood sugar levels, lowering cholesterol, and inhibiting cholesterol absorption. The insoluble fiber absorbs water in the digestive tract to help with elimination, making it a beneficial aid with bowel problems like Crohn's Disease, certain forms of irritable bowel syndrome (IBS), and constipation.

I highly recommend using the Fat Flush protocol food elements in real life, for you, your hubby (or boyfriend), and your kids for all the right health reasons.

THE FAT FLUSH FLAX FACTOR—FEMALES

Flaxseeds are the richest source of a naturally occurring substance known as lignans, which are natural plant-based hormones that have the ability to modulate estrogen levels. Lignans are concentrated 800 times more in whole flaxseeds than in other plants. For those in perimenopause and menopause, the lignans in flaxseeds can have a positive effect on eradicating symptoms like hot flashes and night sweats as well as reducing ovarian dysfunction, balancing menstrual cycle changes, and helping to reduce the risk of osteoporosis by increasing bone density. Some researchers have even observed that the beneficial effects of lignans match those of Tamoxifen, the anticancer drug used for breast cancer.

THE FAT FLUSH FLAX FACTOR—KIDS

Perhaps the best news about flax is its positive effect on children.

Essential fatty acids contained in flaxseed oil and flaxseeds have a dramatic impact on health and vitality throughout our lives, beginning with the development of the infant brain. Over half the brain (60 percent, to be exact) is composed of fat. Brain chemicals known as neurotransmitters are regulated by tissuelike hormones or prostaglandins which are produced by the essential fatty acids. The brain—and the entire nervous system, for that matter—needs the right kind of fats for nourishment and protection.

I strongly suspect that the previous three generations of American kids have not been eating the right kinds of fats for the development of the brain. Could this be a reason why we have so many kids diagnosed with attention deficit hyperactivity disorder (ADHD)?

Our kids are being diagnosed right and left with ADHD and are being prescribed the drug Ritalin. Do you really think our kids are suffering from an epidemic Ritalin deficiency? A growing body of research shows that these children are really suffering from an essential fatty acid deficiency because the clinical signs of such a deficiency match those of ADHD, such as the inability to focus, a short attention span, restlessness, irritability, mood swings, and even panic attacks. Numerous studies over the past two decades have confirmed that kids with ADHD have lower omega-3 levels in their blood than do normal children. When children diagnosed with ADHD start eating the right kinds of fats, many parents notice that their children become calmer and more focused.

This is why you will see recipes for all phases that include foods that the whole family (and especially the kids) will enjoy. The Flaxy Butter Spread (page 216) and Flaxy Syrup (page 218) have been designed with your kids' health in mind.

The final new additions for phases 1 and 2 are ones you will be most thankful for because now you can actually make scrambled eggs without your eggs sticking to the pan.

All Phases New Legal Cheat. Nonstick cooking sprays made primarily from olive oil (like Pam) are the latest, greatest legal cheat. Keep this top secret, please. Use only one 3-second spray to coat the pan and prevent sticking (you scrambled egg lovers will be most appreciative of this, I'm sure).

Another All Phases New Legal Cheat. You now have the option to enjoy 1 cup of a rich, dark, full-bodied caffeine-free herbal coffee (like Teeccino) or 1 cup of dandelion root tea as an alternative to the morning cup of organic coffee.

Flush Flash. Dandelion root tea is a therapeutic tea that helps to clean out both liver and gallbladder congestion. This can be very helpful for those who have taxed their livers by ingesting excessive alcohol, taking the Pill (or other medications), and especially for those taking cholesterol-lowering medications (Lipitor) or acetaminophen-containing Tylenol, Vicodin, or Darvocet. Available in tea or capsule form, at least 1 cup a day is a must for those who are liver-challenged. (See Chapter 14.)

Dandelion roots can also be made into an herbal coffee substitute which is also a great liver tonic.

One More All Phases New Legal Cheat. For those with low blood pressure or chronic fatigue, a pinch of salt is now acceptable for breakfast, lunch, and dinner.

PHASE 2: THE ONGOING FAT FLUSH

Phase 2 friendly carbs now include more colorful and satisfying personal favorites like 1 small yam and 1/2 cup cooked turnips, rutabaga, and parsnips, all of which will make the Plan and the recipes even easier for you to follow with more practical and realistic choices for long-term satisfaction.

You can now choose between 1 slice of Ezekiel 4:9 bread or 1 Ezekiel 4:9 tortilla. Although the tortilla has more carbs (24 carb grams vs. 15 in the bread), it does provide a nice alternative that gets your creative juices going. Many Fat Flushers have shared with me that they use the tortilla to roll up their scrambled eggs in the morning. They drizzle their morning flaxseed oil on the tortilla for extra Fat Flushing goodness.

In addition to zesty turmeric, phase 2 has some other delightful new spices to please your palate that are now Fat Flush friendly. These are Chinese Five Spice powder, rosemary, mint, prepared Dijon mustard, oregano, and basil, formerly only Lifestyle options. The Chinese Five Spice powder, which contains anise, cinnamon, fennel, cloves, and ginger, gives food a sweet, slightly licoricelike flavor, which allows you to satisfy your sweet tooth healthfully and keeps you on the Plan. Rosemary, with its pinelike spice scent and flavor, is good for circulation and memory, and it relieves upset stomachs. Just a mere teaspoon of the crushed leaves can do the trick. Cool and refreshing mint is a powerful flavor booster good for digestion, Dijon mustard helps to rev up metabolism, while robust, pungent oregano is making headlines these days as a natural antibiotic. In fact, the *Journal of Agricultural and Food Chemistry* reported that oregano was the herb highest in antioxidants out of over 25 culinary and medicinal herbs evaluated. The antioxidant potential in oregano is even higher than it is in vitamin E. (Marjoram came in second, by the way.) Basil, with its sweet, clovelike flavor, is a natural antiviral. So, Fat Flush is good for your total health, not just your waistline!

Phases 2 and 3 Flash. If you prefer, you can continue with phase 1 cranwater and the phase 1 recipe for the Long Life Cocktail. These would replace the water recommendation and the new phases 2 and 3 recipe for the Long Life Cocktail.

PHASE 3: THE LIFESTYLE EATING PLAN

The most exciting and innovative news of all for food lovers is that phase 3 has been markedly expanded to include a subsection for special occasions. This section includes new sweetening options for recipes that will make holiday and birthday celebrations more Fat Flush–friendly dessert-wise. You will find modest amounts of date sugar (a great source of minerals like potassium, made from pulverized dates found in health food stores), blackstrap molasses (exceptionally rich in calcium and iron), maple syrup, and even natural, unheated honey as a sweetening choice in the phase 3 special occasions recipes found in the dessert chapter, Nourishing Sweets and Indulgences.

In addition, for those special occasions, you may now enjoy condiment-size portions (notice the word *condiment* here) of dried fruits (like dried figs, dates, raisins or currants, dried plums or prunes, and apricots) as well as some tropical delights that many of you have been craving, like mango and papaya. New fats for special occasions' entertaining and enjoyment now include 1 cup of coconut milk, 2 tablespoons of heavy cream, or 4 tablespoons of whipped cream.

You may be really shocked to see coconut milk on this list. Don't be. You see, despite the coconut's "bad" saturated-fat reputation, it provides strong antiviral protection and adds full-bodied taste and flavor for those company dishes. And I am such a strong believer in the coconut's natural antibiotic virtues (it is also antimicrobial) that I have included 1 tablespoon of unsweetened coconut in your bonus foods listing, along with nuts, avocado, nut butters, butter, cream cheese, mayo, and sour cream, as itemized in the phase 3 lifestyle eating protocol from *The Fat Flush Plan*.

But do keep in mind that while many of these "forbidden" ingredients are now considered Fat Flush–friendly for "special occasions," feel free to offer your kids and your hubby these specialty items and treats—frequently! My guess is that the recipes you will find throughout the book where Phase 3 special occasion recipes are featured (and especially in the Nourishing Sweets and Indulgences chapter) are a whole lot more healthy (and just as tasty, I think) than current white flour, white sugar, trans-fats-laden fast foods and goodies.

And there's even more good news: For everyday phase 3 lifestyle eating, there is a greater selection of fat-flushing foods in the fruits, dairy, and friendly carb categories. For example, 1/2 cup of pineapple (rich in beneficial digestive enzymes) and 12 large grapes (high in the antioxidant resveratrol, helpful in lowering your risk of heart disease) are new refreshing options for phase 3 lifestyle fruit choices. The only caveat here is to keep in mind that if you are still yeast-prone, then the higher-sugar foods like pineapple and grapes should still be omitted. New dairy options now include whole milk yogurt and Parmesan and Romano cheese (good for topping off veggie dishes and salads).

You may be pleasantly surprised to note that some familiar old friends are now Fat Flush–friendly. These newly added friendly carbs include beets (naturally good liver cleansers), oatmeal (rich in a cholesterol-lowering fiber known as beta-glucan), nutty wheat germ (high in vitamin E and folic acid) and even chestnuts, because they are delicious and good for the soul. Please note that although both oatmeal and wheat germ contain very small amounts of gluten, they are usually tolerated well by phase 3, especially when used in moderation and rotated into the diet plan.

The special occasion friendly carbs represent the most desirable carbohydrate choices for thickening and baking purposes that are in line with the Fat Flush philosophy of healthy fats and being moderate to low on the glycemic index. The special occasion friendly carbs also boast a fairly low carbohydrate count in comparison to whole grain flours as well as to rice flour and corn meal. Moderate amounts of almond meal, for example, are featured in some of the recipes, and I invite you to be creative with these new special occasion choices.

Phase 3 herbs and spices have been extended, as you will be gratified and perhaps grateful to see. There are special occasion flavor enhancers you will savor (like some wheat-free low-sodium tamari that you might have once in a while) plus a consolidated list of legal extras. Finally, you will certainly be very happy to note that various types of alcohol are allowed for those Phase 3 special occasions. At around 200°F, alcohol burns off, leaving a delightful flavor and only 15 percent of the original calories.

Because the phase 3 updates are more expansive, here's a more detailed overview of the latest food options. I must remind you, once again, that these listings are incomplete—so please do refer to *The Fat Flush Plan* for the basic phase 3 protocols, upon which these brand-new additions build.

Additional Bonus Food. 1 tablespoon of unsweetened coconut.

New Special Occasion Fats. These can be used in place of 2 tablespoons of daily oil. **Choose from** 1 cup of coconut milk, 2 tablespoons of heavy cream, or 4 tablespoons of whipped cream.

Health Tip. Despite the coconut's "bad" saturated-fat reputation, it provides strong antiviral protection and adds full-bodied taste and flavor for those company dishes.

Special Occasion Fruits, Juices, and Sweeteners. These can be used in place of one or more portions of phase 3 fruit. **Choose from** 1 large dried fig, 2 dates, 2 tablespoons raisins or currants, 2 dried plums or prunes, 3 dried apricot halves, 1/2 cup unsweetened apple sauce, 1/2 small mango, 1/3 medium papaya, 1 tablespoon date sugar, 1 tablespoon blackstrap molasses, 1 tablespoon honey, 1 tablespoon maple syrup, 2 tablespoons unsweetened fruit preserves of any kind, and 1/2 cup unsweetened juice.

These natural sweeteners are high in vitamins and minerals (like vitamin A, potassium, calcium, and iron) and also stand up well to heat in recipes. The healthiest dried fruits are those that are unsulfured. Sulfur-based compounds are vitamin B destroyers and in certain individuals can create allergic reactions.

Insider Tip. Date sugar is available from Bob's Red Mill. Knudsen, Mountain Sun, and Lakewood carry unsweetened fruit juices.

Dairy. Additional phase 3 choices include 1 cup of whole milk yogurt, 2 percent cottage cheese, or 4 tablespoons of Parmesan or Romano cheese.

Friendly Carbohydrates. Additional phase 3 choices include 1/2 cup of beets, 1/2 cup steel cut or old-fashioned rolled oats, 3 tablespoons of wheat germ, and 4 large chestnuts.

Insider Tip. If bloating gas or weight gain is noted, omit the new carb serving and revert to the diet of the previous week. After the symptoms have subsided, add back 1/4 cup (or other incremental amounts) of a different carbohydrate and monitor your response until you reach your tolerance level.

Special Occasion Friendly Carbohydrates. These can be used in place of one or more servings of carbs as part of your friendly carb daily intake. Special occasion choices include 1/2 cup of almond meal.

Fat-Flushing Herbs and Spices. Additional phase 3 choices include other flavorful spices, herbs, and condiments like allspice, cardamom, nutmeg, saffron, marjoram, and horseradish.

Special Occasion Flavor Enhancers. A touch of low-sodium Tamari (wheat-free soy sauce), wine, vermouth, sherry, rum, or Pernod can be used in phase 3 recipes. When the alcohol is used for cooking, most of it is burned off while the flavor remains. Alcohol burnoff takes about a half hour when food is simmering in soups and stews. It burns off in 3 minutes when used to sauté. Try to avoid "cooking wine," which contains added salt. The term *cooking wine* refers to an earlier time when wine set aside for use in food was purposefully salted to prevent the cook from drinking it.

Legal Extras. Cocoa powder, carob powder, flavor extracts (vanilla, anise, almond, lemon, mint, rum, or orange).

Special Occasion Baking Needs. Aluminum-free baking powder (Royal, Rumford, Price, or Schillings).

Do note that *The Fat Flush Kit* from Uni Key Health Systems contains all the recommended dietary supplement formulas for all phases. (See Chapter 14.)

3 The Fat Flush Kitchen

Cooking the Fat Flush way is easy when you are well equipped with the tools of the trade. In addition to a selection of herbs and spices for revving up your metabolism, powering up your health, and tickling your taste buds, there are some basic Fat Flush–friendly cooking utensils that merit your consideration. Utensils like waterless cookware and high-quality knives are a lifetime investment in health and well-being. Following is a list of very basic equipment for your Fat Flush kitchen.

ESSENTIAL UTENSILS

Although many of the recipes in this book call for a nonstick skillet or baking sheet, you may want to consider using heavy-duty, stainless steel, waterless cookware, which cooks food in a vacuum seal. When food cooks in its own juices, high flavor, tenderness, and high nutritional value are guaranteed. In fact, studies have shown that cooking in vacuum-sealed cookware rather than nonsealed cookware retains more vitamins and minerals and produces less fat. At the same time, less salt and less of every seasoning is required for high-quality taste. I personally use Le Creuset cookware for all my cooking. Although it is a heavier line of cookware, I feel secure that it is enamel covered iron and safe.

Enamel, Corning Ware, glass, and Pyrex are also acceptable. For those of you who are anemic, you might consider cooking with iron-based utensils because the extra iron picked up from cooking can actually be therapeutic. When a high acid-based food like spaghetti sauce, for example, is cooked in iron pots, it contains six times more iron than when it is made in ceramic cookware.

Choose nonstick, heavy-duty tin or black steel for your baking needs.

STAY AWAY FROM ALUMINUM

Aluminum-proof the kitchen as much as possible. Aluminum inhibits the body's utilization of key minerals like magnesium, calcium, and phosphorus. Some researchers believe that it can neutralize pepsin, an important digestive enzyme in the stomach. Replace all aluminum steamers, measuring cups, spoons, bread pans, and cookie sheets with stainless steel, high-quality plastic, or Pyrex.

You should avoid aluminum foil also. When cooking, opt for parchment paper (like Beyond Gourmet unbleached parchment paper), which the French have used for years in their fish "en papillote" dishes to seal in juices. This can be used for roasting veggies as well. For storing and freezing, you can first cover with wax paper and then foil, which prevents the aluminum from leaching into foods.

CURB THE COPPER

You would also be wise to replace all copper-lined cookware. This metal has an affinity for Vitamin C and can upset the sensitive zinc/copper balance in your system. Excess copper has been linked to depression, insomnia, anorexia nervosa, compulsive behavior, anxiety, hyperactivity, various skin disorders, and hair loss. Need I say more?

CONSIDER A WATER
FILTER FOR YOUR HOME

With pure, clean water becoming extinct and bottled water not always reliable, a home water filter is no longer a luxury but a necessity. I recommend the Doulton Ceramic Water Filter, the most effective water filtration system available. The filter is made of ultrafine ceramic with pores so small that they trap bacteria, parasites, and particles down to 0.5 microns in size. The filtering system provides a comprehensive, three-stage process. In the first stage the tiny pores in the ceramic remove bacteria, parasites, and rust and dirt. The second filter stage is composed of high-density matrix carbon that removes chlorine, pesticides, and other chemicals. In the third stage, a heavy metal-removing compound eliminates lead and copper. (See Chapter 14.)

KNIVES

I would be very remiss if I did not remind you how important the right knives are for chopping, paring, slicing, and carving—everything from fruits and veggies to roasts and turkeys. At the very least, you will need at least one high-quality utility knife and one 4-inch paring knife for the majority of your cutting needs in the Fat Flush kitchen. If you are planning to purchase a new knife set and you want it to be durable, then I highly recommend MAC Japanese knives, which are acclaimed by chefs all over the world as the world's finest knives. The MAC knives are what I personally use because they have a razor sharp edge, stay sharp a long time, and have thin blades for easy slicing. (See Chapter 14.)

THERMOS COOKER

A wide-mouthed thermos is helpful for taking soups, stews, and leftovers to work with you.

THE FLAXSEED GRINDER

Since ground up flaxseeds are such a potent source of the metabolism-boosting omega-3s and fiber-rich lignans, which function as natural hormone balancers, a specially designed flaxseed grinder is a valuable Fat Flush kitchen item. I have discovered the Ultimate Flaxseed Grinder with three settings and push button controls. (See Chapter 14.)

MORTAR AND PESTLE

Many of the recipes call for crushed dried herbs. A mortar and pestle is best for extracting the essence of the dried herbs and spices used in the recipes. The mortar and pestle crushes the herbs which in turn releases the volatile oils that contain the herbs' health and aromatic qualities. The aromas of the ground dried herbs or spices are nearly four times as strong as the same herbs and spices before they are ground.

SEED GRINDER

For grinding and crushing seeds (like anise, fennel, or coriander), a small hand-turned mill is very useful.

THE THRILL OF THE GRILL:
GAS VERSUS CHARCOAL

Grilling is here to stay. And nothing says outdoor fun more than a cook-out. Many Fat Flush recipes from the delicious main course lamb and fish kebabs to snacks featuring various seasonal fruit kebabs make use of a grill. Healthwise, the oxidative reaction of charcoal grilling (a combination of browning and charring) may be somewhat toxic. Food can soak up added chemicals from the charcoal briquettes, too. So if you are a charcoal fan, then please be sure to cut off any charred, burned, or blackened portions of food.

Gas grilling is another way to go, especially if there is no sensitivity to hydrocarbons which are the by-products of gas combustion. Healthier or not, most grill owners seem to prefer gas grills because they are easier to light. To compensate for the smoky flavor that charcoal imparts, many gas grill owners use natural wood chips from hickory, mesquite, or oak.

The safest way to protect your food from harmful substances formed during the grilling process is to marinate, marinate, marinate. Some research shows that marinades can cut down on carcinogen production by nearly 99 percent.

Marinade Tip. In the phase 3 lifestyle program, you can make some easy grilling marinades by combining about 1 cup of olive oil, 1/2 cup of fresh lime or lemon juice, and 1/4 cup of cider vinegar seasoned with some of your favorite herbs. For special occasions, this basic marinade can be jazzed up with a tablespoon of date sugar or honey.

OTHER HELPFUL FAT FLUSH
KITCHEN EQUIPMENT

Food processor/blender for whipping up smoothies and pâtés
Toaster oven

HELPFUL FAT FLUSH COOKWARE

Nonstick skillets and saucepans (various sizes)
Stainless steel steamer
Dutch oven, 3 1/2 quart or 6 quart slow cooker or Crock Pot

HELPFUL FAT FLUSH BAKEWARE

Ramekins
Nonstick baking sheets
Oven-proof baking dishes
Casseroles

HELPFUL FAT FLUSH COOKING TOOLS AND CUTLERY

Wooden spoons
Measuring spoons
Measuring cups
Slotted spoon
2 chopping boards (1 for meats, 1 for veggies)
Rubber spatulas
Mixing bowls (various sizes)
Lemon juicer
Tongs
Pastry brush for basting
Garlic press
Grater
Can opener
Scissors
Ceramic sharpening rod
Masher
Whisk
Popsicle molds
Freezer-proof, airtight containers
Grilling accessories (broad-headed jumbo tongs and turner tongs with
    one-sided spatula)

FAT FLUSH INGREDIENT EQUIVALENTS

WHEN YOU DON'T HAVE	YOU CAN USE
Garlic, 1 clove, fresh	1/8 teaspoon garlic powder
Gingerroot, 1 teaspoon, grated, fresh	1/4 teaspoon ground ginger
Herb, 1 tablespoon, fresh	1/2 to 1 teaspoon dried herb, crushed
Herb, 1 teaspoon, fresh	1/2 teaspoon dried herb, ground
Onion, 1 small (1/3 cup)	1 teaspoon onion powder or 1 tablespoon dried minced onion
Tomato sauce, 2 cups	3/4 cup tomato paste plus 1 cup water

FAT FLUSH RECIPE MAKEOVERS FOR EVERY DAY AND SPECIAL OCCASIONS

WHEN THE RECIPE CALLS FOR:	YOU CAN USE INSTEAD (IF APPROPRIATE TO YOUR PHASE):
1 tablespoon brown sugar	1 tablespoon date sugar (If used in baking, this is best added toward the end to prevent burning. Adding water to the date sugar to make a syrup consistency will also work.)
1 tablespoon sugar	1 teaspoon Flora-Key, 1 1/2 packets Stevia Plus or 1/2 tablespoon honey, molasses, or pure maple syrup
1 cup sugar for baking	1/2 cup honey (If you are using as much as 3/4 cup honey, then decrease other liquids by 1/4 cup for each 3/4 cup honey. If there is no liquid in recipe, then add 1/4 cup flaxseed meal for each 3/4 cup honey. Also, lower the baking temperature to a maximum of 250°F; both honey and molasses tend to caramelize at higher temperatures.)

1 ounce or 1 square baking chocolate	3 tablespoons carob powder plus 1 tablespoon water plus 1 tablespoon sesame or rice bran oil
Breading	Fat Flush Bread Crumbs (page 203) or ground flaxseeds. (Keep in mind that cooking with ground flaxseeds above 300°F can damage the seeds' oil and covert it into the unhealthy trans form, but the lignans will not be damaged at high heat.)
Sauce and soup thickeners	Thicken Thin—not starch thickener (*www.expertfoods.com*)—for sauces, soups, and gravies
1 tablespoon margarine or cooking oil	1 tablespoon butter or 3 tablespoons ground flaxseed. (Either shorten the baking time or lower oven temperature by 25°F because baked goods will brown more quickly with flaxseed.)

FAT FLUSH EQUIVALENTS CHART FOR DRY MEASUREMENTS

Multiply ounces by 28 to convert into grams
Multiply pounds by .45 to convert into kilograms
Multiply grams by .035 to convert into ounces
Multiply kilograms by 2.2 to convert into pounds

FAT FLUSH EQUIVALENTS FOR LIQUID MEASUREMENTS

Multiply ounces by 30 to convert into milliliters
Multiply pints by .47 to convert into liters
Multiply quarts by .95 to convert into liters
Multiply gallons by 3.8 to convert into liters
Multiply milliliters by 0.34 to convert into ounces

FAT FLUSH EQUIVALENTS CHART

U.S.	METRIC
1/8 teaspoon	0.5 milliliter
1/4 teaspoon	1 milliliter
1/2 teaspoon	2 milliliters
1 teaspoon	5 milliliters
1 tablespoon	1 tablespoon
1/4 cup or 2 fluid ounces	60 milliliters
1/3 cup or 3 fluid ounces	80 milliliters
1/2 cup or 4 fluid ounces	120 milliliters
2/3 cup or 5 fluid ounces	160 milliliters
3/4 cup or 6 fluid ounces	180 milliliters
1 cup or 8 fluid ounces	240 milliliters
11/4 cups	1 cup
2 cups	1 pint
1 quart	1 liter
1/2 inch	1.27 centimeter
1 inch	2.54 centimeter

HANDY INFORMATION EQUIVALENTS

8 drops = a dash
1/3 of 1/2 teaspoon = a pinch
3 teaspoons = 1 tablespoon
2 tablespoons (liquid) = 1 ounce
4 tablespoons = 1/4 cup
51/3 tablespoons = 1/3 cup
8 tablespoons = 1/2 cup
102/3 tablespoons = 2/3 cup
16 tablespoons = 1 cup
1/8 cup = 2 tablespoons
1/3 cup = 5 tablespoons plus 1 teaspoon
2/3 cup = 10 tablespoons plus 2 teaspoons
8 fluid ounces = 1 cup
16 fluid ounces = 2 cups = 1 pint
2 pints = 1 quart
4 cups = 1 quart
4 quarts = 1 gallon

FAT FLUSH BAKING PAN SIZES

U.S.	METRIC
8-inch by 1½-inch pan	20-centimeter by 4-centimeter cake or sandwich tin
9-inch by 1½-inch pan	23-centimeter by 3.5-centimeter cake or sandwich tin
11-inch by 7-inch pan	28-centimeter by 18-centimeter baking tin
13-inch by 9-inch pan	32.5-centimeter by 23-centimeter baking tin
15-inch by 10-inch pan	38-centimeter by 25.5-centimeter baking tin
1½-quart casserole	1.5-liter casserole
2-quart casserole	2-liter casserole
2-quart rectangular baking dish	30-centimeter by 20-centimeter by 3-centimeter baking tin
9-inch pie plate	22-centimeter by 4-centimeter or 23-centimeter by 4-centimeter pie plate
7- or 8-inch springform pan	18-centimeter or 20-centimeter springform or loose bottom cake tin
9-inch by 5-inch loaf pan	23-centimeter by 13-centimeter or 2-pound narrow loaf tin

OVEN TEMPERATURE CONVERSIONS

FAHRENHEIT	CELSIUS	GAS SETTING
300 degrees F	150 degrees C	2
325 degrees F	160 degrees C	3
350 degrees F	180 degrees C	4
375 degrees F	190 degrees C	5
400 degrees F	200 degrees C	6
425 degrees F	220 degrees C	7
450 degrees F	230 degrees C	8
Broil		Grill

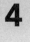 # The Fat Flush Herbs and Spices for Weight Loss and Health

As you may recall from reading *The Fat Flush Plan*, the recommended herbs and spices are much more than simply flavor enhancers. In phase 1, certain seasonings are utilized because they are helpful in boosting metabolism (cayenne, ginger, and mustard), keeping blood sugar levels stable (cinnamon, cloves, and bay leaves), removing fluid from the system (parsley, cilantro, and coriander), nourishing the liver (garlic and turmeric), and aiding digestion (anise, fennel, cumin, and dill). In phase 2, the addition of basil and oregano is helpful for combating germs and viruses, while mint is another natural digestive aid. Rosemary, also a new phase 2 seasoning, acts as a potent antioxidant, helping to protect breast health. Others like phase 3-recommended cardamom, nutmeg, saffron, and marjoram are rich in minerals like potassium, manganese, and iron, and also assist in digestive function.

While fresh herbs are generally preferable to dried ones (with the exception of oregano), as mentioned before it is not always possible to find fresh. But if you do have fresh herbs easily available, they are generally better than the dried for salads and sauces. The dried go best with longer-cooking dishes like stews, soups, and casseroles. The rule of thumb is that 1 teaspoon of dried equals 1 tablespoon of fresh.

Do keep in mind that fresh herbs can be frozen. So whether you buy your herbs in the produce section of your supermarket or grow them yourself (some do quite well right on your windowsill), there is no reason to let them go bad in the fridge or just wilt away. Freeze 'em!

Put the leaves, whether whole or chopped, in small bags and freeze them for future use. And the best part of all is that when you do decide to use your fresh frozen herbs for culinary purposes, you can add them frozen to your cooked dishes. There is no need to defrost them beforehand.

Dried herbs and spices have a shelf life of about six months. After this amount of time, many of them lose their flavor and become flat. So store your herbs and spices in small, airtight jars in a cool, dry, dark place away from the kitchen stove, where heat can affect them. A cool environment protects the volatile oils from warmth and moisture, which can change zesty, aromatic, and pungent flavors.

If you are buying your herbs and spices in stores, try to find nonirradiated herbs and spices such as Frontier Herbs and The Spice Hunter. When you open a jar of dried herbs, there should be a fresh, strong, and distinctive aroma. If there is not—and they also taste like dried grass rather than lovely herbs (this is the truly best way to explain this)—then you won't be deriving the weight loss and health benefits from these herbal helpers. Their full flavor potential will be lost, and it is high time to replace your supply.

Here is a rundown of the main Fat Flush herbs used in this cookbook so you can see at a glance how they have traditionally been used in culinary applications as well as how they can enhance your health at the same time.

Anise
MILDLY AROMATIC

Culinary. Found in whole-seed form. Licoricelike taste is similar to fennel and great for seasoning cabbage, cauliflower, turnips, beef, shellfish, cakes, and cookies. Chewing on a few seeds has a natural breath mintlike effect. Provides a nice touch to teas.

Therapeutic. Helpful for liver, kidneys, and stomach. Enhances lactation. Once considered an aphrodisiac.

Basil
AROMATICALLY ROBUST

A native of India, folklore says it blesses those it touches.

Culinary. Found in fresh, dried-leaf, or flaked form. Leaves are wonderful with any type of tomato dish. Ministrips of fresh basil are great with tomato dishes from sauces to soups. Goes well with sauces, stews, soups, stuffings, and dips. A pesto staple. Frequently found in Mediterranean-style dishes from Italy and Greece. Chopped basil is a special treat with fresh corn on the cob.

Therapeutic. Helps nervous exhaustion, anxiety, colds, depression, substance abuse, and drug withdrawal. Appetite stimulant.

Bay leaf
SEMIMILD TASTE AND AROMA

Keeps bugs out of the cupboard!

Culinary. Found in dried-leaf form. Stronger if the leaves are torn for cooking. Used in soups, chowders, stews, roasts, gravies, and marinades. Remember to remove before eating.

Therapeutic. Known to relieve bronchitis, arthritis, and atherosclerosis. Tones and strengthens digestive tract.

Cardamom
STRONGLY AROMATIC WITH AN AFTERTASTE REMINISCENT OF LEMONS

Culinary. Found in whole or ground form. Highlighted in Indian foods. Goes well with curries, rice, and breads. Especially nice in teas and herbal coffees.

Therapeutic. Helps treat indigestion, asthma, bronchitis, celiac disease, bad breath, spastic colon, and vomiting. Considered an aphrodisiac in the Middle East. Potent digestive aid for grains.

Cayenne
HOT AND SPICY

Culinary. A member of the chili family, found most frequently in ground form. Good with sauces, vegetables, beans, and dips, and in fish and meat dishes. A prime ingredient in Tex-Mex cuisine and Asian types of foods.

Therapeutic. Soothing to irritated tissues. Stimulates circulation, relieves migraines, assists digestion, breaks up congestion, and stimulates the production of adrenal hormones which speed up the breakdown of fat by 25 percent.

Cilantro
MILDLY SPICY

Culinary. Also known as Chinese parsley, cilantro is a fresh herb with a more pungent taste than parsley. It is good with salads, soups, and tomato-based dishes and as a garnish. Frequently found in Mexican food and in Asian cuisine.

Therapeutic. A heavy metal eliminator, cilantro helps relieve bloating, diarrhea, and GI tract disorders.

Cinnamon
SUBTLE, SWEET-SPICY

Cinnamon's scent has been found by the Smell and Taste Research Institute to enhance arousal in males.

Culinary. Very versatile and typically found in stick or ground form. Can be used in lamb, beef, and chicken dishes as well as with fruits, breads,

onions, squash, tomatoes, sweet potatoes, and cereal grains. Good seasoning for teas.

Therapeutic. Helpful for diabetics by making cells more insulin-sensitive,
can boost body's ability to balance blood sugar about twentyfold. Good
for cramps, bloating, and flatulence.

Cloves
HIGHLY AROMATIC AND SWEET

Culinary. Whole or in ground form, cloves are good for adding spice to
stewed fruit and character to roasts, sweet potatoes, and wild game.
Lovely for seasoning teas.

Therapeutic. Acts as a parasite fighter, also aids in relieving diarrhea, sore
throats, toothaches, and stomach cramps.

Coriander
MODERATELY SPICY WITH A HINT OF ORANGE PEEL

Coriander actually comes from the seeds of the cilantro plant. I have a per-
fume called Coriandre from Paris that I absolutely adore and that has
become my signature scent.

Culinary. Found in seed or ground form, coriander is a favorite in Latin
American and Indian curry-based dishes. Excellent seasoning for carrots,
fish, chicken, eggs, beans, and rice.

Therapeutic. Treats bloating, cramps, and GI disorders.

Cumin
DISTINCTIVELY SPICY WITH EARTHY, MEATY FLAVOR

Culinary. Found in seed or ground form in Middle Eastern, East Indian,
African, and Mexican cuisine. Good with beans, dips, stews, lamb, beef,
and sauces.

Therapeutic. Improves liver function and relieves gas, colic, and digestive-
connected headaches.

Dill
MILDLY AROMATIC

Culinary. Found in fresh, seed, or dried form. Featured in Northern and
Eastern European cooking. Enhances fish dishes, cucumbers, beans,

salads, cabbage, soup, salad dressings, cottage cheese, egg dishes, and tofu dips.

Therapeutic. Helpful for indigestion, colic, bad breath, and insomnia.

Fennel
MILD TASTE AND AROMA

Culinary. Found in fresh, dried-leaf, or seed form. The distinctive licorice-like taste goes well with fish, turkey, cabbage, onions, tomato sauces, and stews. Provides a nice touch for cookies and cakes (healthy ones, of course).

Therapeutic. Helpful as a natural digestive aid and as a phytoestrogen. Good for bad breath, diabetes, kidney stones, and nausea.

Garlic
PUNGENT
THE KING OF THE HERBS

Culinary. Found in fresh, powdered, or minced form. Garlic is featured in worldwide cuisines especially for fish, poultry, game, vegetables, soups, beans, salsas, salad dressings, casseroles, and marinades.

Therapeutic. Most potent healthwise when garlic is mashed, smashed, or minced raw. Helps to protect against heart disease, asthma, diabetes, flu, and stomach cancer. Garlic is the best antiparasitic, antifungal, and antiyeast herb.

Ginger
HOT, PUNGENT, AND WARMING

Culinary. Found in fresh, whole-root, or ground form. Highlighted in Chinese and Indian spice mixtures. Perks up meats, marinades, root vegetables, fruits, cookies, and cakes.

Therapeutic. Good for motion sickness, muscle soreness, arthritis, headaches, poor circulation, flatulence, and menstrual cramps. Serves as a natural blood thinner and anti-inflammatory.

Horseradish
PUNGENT

Culinary. Fresh root or dried in powdered form. Great addition to dips, meatloaf, egg dishes, and sauces.

Therapeutic. Helpful for relieving sinus congestion and clearing excess mucus and phlegm.

Marjoram
SWEET MARJORAM IS FRAGRANT AND FLAVORFUL. A MILDER RELATIVE
OF OREGANO. ALSO USED IN PERFUMES!

Culinary. Found in fresh or dried, leaf form. Featured in Greek, French, and Italian cooking, sweet marjoram is a nice addition to sauces, soups, stews, stuffings, and salads.

Therapeutic. Relieves menstrual cramps and bronchitis, calms nerves, and is helpful for insomnia.

Mint
MILDLY AROMATIC

Culinary. Found in fresh or dried-leaf form. Perfect for lamb, peas, salads, lentils, and beverages.

Therapeutic. Helps relieve flatulence, fatigue, gallbladder problems, morning sickness, and nausea. Acts as a parasite fighter, antimicrobial, and digestive aid.

Mustard
MODERATELY SPICY

Culinary. Found in whole-seed or ground form. Used with egg dishes like deviled eggs. Also used with meat, sauces, dips, condiments, salad dressings, marinades, and shellfish.

Therapeutic. Increases body's fat-burning ability, raises body temperature, acts as a diuretic, and increases circulation.

Nutmeg
WARMING, POWERFUL, AND SWEET

Culinary. Found in whole or ground form. Most pungent when grated fresh at the end of cooking. Used to infuse soups, sauces, cheese and shellfish dishes. Goes well with spinach and cauliflower.

Therapeutic. A natural digestive aid, nutmeg relieves flatulence and coughs and reduces pain.

Oregano
PUNGENT AND MILDLY SPICY
CONTAINS HIGHEST AMOUNT OF ANTIOXIDANTS IN THE HERB KINGDOM.

Culinary. Found in fresh or dried-leaf form. Best when added toward the end of cooking, or it can become bitter. A staple of Italian and Mediterranean cooking, oregano seasons tomatoes, vegetables, salad dressings, and sauces.

Therapeutic. A well-respected antibacterial, antiviral, anti-inflammatory, and antioxidant, oregano relieves candida, nausea, colic, bronchitis, and motion sickness.

Parsley
MILD TASTE AND AROMA

Culinary. Found in fresh or dried-leaf form. This is one herb in which the dried form is not at all flavorful. Most flavorful when fresh parsley is added near the end of cooking. Complements all cuisine, especially salads, soups, tofu dishes, soufflés, dips, and pâtés.

Therapeutic. Great natural diuretic and helps to treat problems with kidneys, gout, anemia, jaundice, and arthritis.

Rosemary
PUNGENTLY SPICY

Culinary. Found in fresh or dried-leaf form. Great with Italian dishes, lamb, chicken, marinades, and casseroles and as flavoring for bread.

Therapeutic. Potent antioxidant, energy booster, relieves upset stomach, and good for the memory and hair.

Sage
SHARP, SPICY, AND HIGHLY AROMATIC
THE AMERICAN INDIANS USED SAGE TO SMUDGE AWAY EVIL SPIRITS.

Culinary. Found in fresh or dried-leaf form. Goes well with stuffing, poultry, onions, peas, cottage cheese, casseroles, sauces, and omelets.

Therapeutic. A natural phytoestrogen, sage is helpful as a menopause remedy and also helps to stimulate and regulate the flow of bile so it is good with fatty foods. It is a decongestant, gargle, and astringent (natural deodorants use sage), and it treats fevers, colds, and flu.

Tarragon
MILD AND AROMATIC

Culinary. Found in fresh or dried-leaf form. A favorite of French cooks, tarragon's delicate flavor enhances chicken, fish, and seafood. Good for salad dressings and with apple cider vinegar.

Therapeutic. Helps to eliminate parasites in children, acts like a natural diuretic, and supports digestive function.

Thyme
DELICATE AND AROMATIC

Culinary. Found in fresh or dried-leaf form. Goes well with stuffing, soups, sauces, stews, peas, and lentils.

Therapeutic. A natural antibiotic, good for asthma, colds, colic, hangovers, hay fever, headaches, and cough. Helps with digestion of fatty foods.

Turmeric
MILDLY SPICY

Culinary. This yellowish relative of ginger is a fat digestant. Most commonly used with curries, beans, and fish dishes and in scrambled tofu.

Therapeutic. Packed with anticancer antioxidants, turmeric contains curcumin which helps the body detoxify harmful chemicals. Treats arthritis and stops food poisoning, especially salmonella.

Fat Flush Bonus Tip: Learn the art of herbal infusions! Herbed vinegars are Fat Flush friendly for all phases, depending upon the herbs you choose. For example, in phase 1, you could fill up a clean jar or glass bottle with about 1 cup of fresh herbs such as dill or parsley and add 1 quart of cider vinegar. In phase 2, you might choose basil or rosemary, and in phase 3, tarragon or thyme. Cover the bottle. Let this stand in your pantry or some other cool, dark place and, if you wish, after a few days, add even more vinegar. Let stand for another 3 to 4 weeks, and you have a ready-made salad dressing accompaniment or a steamed veggie pick-me-up.

Fat Flush Bonus Tip: In phase 3, you can make an olive, grape seed, or sesame seed infusion by filling up a glass jar with 3 tablespoons of fresh herbs (make sure you pound them slightly to help release the volatile oils and flavor). Then add 1/2 cup of lightly warmed oil of your choice. Let the oil cool, seal the jar, and place it in the fridge for a couple of weeks before you are ready to serve. What a treat on steamed veggies, salads, or brown rice!

5 Breakfast

Breakfast is clearly *the* most important meal of the day. While every one of these phase 1 breakfasts can be enjoyed in each consecutive phase, those recipes specific to phases 2 and 3 are clearly identified below.

The Fat Flush smoothies and egg dishes are a great way to get you going. They can be whipped up in a flash and are a tasty example of meals in minutes. The high protein content of the breakfast recipes (eggs, whey, turkey, tofu, cheese) will rev up your metabolism, the quality fats (like flaxseed oil) will keep you satisfied for hours, while the fruits and veggies impart wholesome energy in the form of slow-acting carbohydrates.

As in all the recipes, it is really the aroma of fresh herbs and spices (delicate dill, pungent cilantro, zesty cayenne) and flavor extracts (vanilla, mint, orange) that make these dishes and smoothies memorable. Do keep in mind that even though many of the recipes call for dried herbs, you can always use fresh if available.

SMOOTHIES

EGGS 'N' SUCH

BREAD AND CEREAL

SMOOTHIES

Tofruity Smoothie

Many Fat Flushers are vegetarians who are big tofu fans. Tofu makes the shake extra creamy. Enjoy this Tofruity Smoothie as part of the plan's twice-a-week soy allowance.

4   ounces extra-firm tofu
1   cup berries, frozen, or fruit of choice from phase 1
1   cup purified water
1   serving whey protein powder
1   tablespoon flaxseed oil
     Stevia Plus to taste

Combine all ingredients in blender. Mix until rich and creamy, about 2–3 minutes.

Enjoy!

Variation:
Try substituting your 1 cup of Teeccino for the 1 cup of water for an interesting taste treat.

ALL PHASES; SERVES 1

Fruit Smoothie

Here is the foundation for your fast-food breakfasts—Fat Flush style. Many of my readers enjoy a second smoothie midafternoon for a quick pick-me-up. Make sure to adjust your fruit intake accordingly.

1 cup fruit, fresh or frozen (strawberries, raspberries, blueberries, or frozen peaches or 1 fresh peach)
1 serving whey protein powder
8 ounces (1 cup) cran-water or plain purified water
1 tablespoon flaxseed oil
¼ teaspoon Stevia Plus, or to taste

Combine all ingredients in blender. Mix until rich and creamy, about 2–3 minutes.

Enjoy!

Variations:
• *For phase 2:* try 1/2 teaspoon crushed mint with any acceptable fruit.
• *For phase 3:* try a dash of nutmeg and ginger with strawberries or 1/2 a frozen banana. (Ripe bananas are great for freezing, by the way, and create a frosty smoothie.)

ALL PHASES; SERVES 1

Very Berry Smoothie

Here is an interesting variation on the smoothie theme. The Stevia Plus works well to take the edge off of the tartness of the cranberries.

3/4   cup raspberries, frozen
1/4   cup cranberries
1   cup purified water
1/4   teaspoon Stevia Plus
1   serving whey protein powder
1   cup ice cubes
1   tablespoon flaxseed oil

Combine all ingredients in blender. Mix until rich and creamy, about 2–3 minutes.

Enjoy!

Variation:

Try substituting 1/2 or 1 small pomegranate for the cranberries, and omit the Stevia Plus.

ALL PHASES; SERVES 1

Super Smoothie

This idea was inspired by Nancy Rodriquez, who lost 15 pounds and still count-ing after just two weeks! She creatively combined the Long Life Cocktail with the smoothie to make this souped-up Super Smoothie. You can use any berry of your choice.

8   ounces (1 cup) cran-water
¼   cup cranberries, fresh or frozen
¾   cup blueberries, frozen
1   serving whey protein powder
1   tablespoon flaxseed oil
1   tablespoon flaxseeds, ground
    Stevia Plus to taste

Combine all ingredients in blender. Mix until rich and creamy, about 2–3
    minutes.

Enjoy!

ALL PHASES; SERVES 1

Pineapple Orange Smoothie

Here's an early morning taste treat. The wheat germ is a good source of heart healthy vitamin E. Just remember that 3 tablespoons of toasted wheat germ is the equivalent of 1 slice of Ezekiel 4:9 toast.

1	cup plain yogurt
½	cup crushed pineapple
3	tablespoons toasted wheat germ
½	cup purified water
1	cup ice cubes
¼–½	teaspoon orange extract

Combine all ingredients in blender. Mix until rich and creamy, about 2–3 minutes.

Enjoy!

PHASE 3; SERVES 1

Super Phase 3 Smoothie

Rose Grandy created this recipe for those mornings when you need more than just a simple smoothie. The calcium rich yogurt and fiber are filling. The cranberries, strawberries, and raspberries are rich in antioxidants and vitamin C—good for your arteries and heart.

8   ounces (1 cup) cran-water
1/4 cup cranberries, fresh or frozen
3/4 cup mixed strawberries and raspberries
1   serving whey protein powder
1   tablespoon flaxseed oil
1   teaspoon powdered psyllium husks or 1 tablespoon flaxseeds,
     ground
1   cup plain yogurt
     Stevia Plus to taste

Combine all ingredients in blender. Mix until rich and creamy, about 2–3
    minutes.

Enjoy!

PHASE 3; SERVES 1

Dandy Strawberry Smoothie

The whole family could enjoy this one without even knowing how healthy it is. But first, double the recipe and try it on your hubby!

1   cup plain yogurt
1   cup strawberries, frozen
1   cup Dandelion Root Tea or Coffee, brewed and chilled
1   serving whey protein powder
    Stevia Plus to taste
1   tablespoon flaxseed oil

Combine all ingredients in blender. Mix until rich and creamy, about 2–3 minutes.

Enjoy!

Phase 3; Serves 1

EGGS 'N' SUCH

Peppers and Egg Scrambler

Colorful and quick, how about a little Homemade Salsa (recipe on page 207) to top if off?

½ cup green pepper, chopped
½ cup red pepper, chopped
¼ cup onion, chopped
¼ cup no-salt-added chicken broth or 1-2-3 Chicken Broth (page 222)
8 eggs
¼ cup purified water

In a medium skillet over medium heat, cook peppers and onions in broth until tender. Beat eggs and water until foamy and pour over the vegetables. As mixture starts to set, gently slide pancake turner across bottom and sides of pan, creating soft curds. Reduce heat to low and continue cooking until eggs are set. Serve immediately.

ALL PHASES; SERVES 4

Eggs Florentine à la Cumin

The cumin in this recipe imparts a nutty taste and Middle Eastern touch. And, of course, the spinach in the recipe is so good for you because it is brimming with heart-smart folic acid.

1 cup chopped spinach (fresh or thawed, drained and patted dry)
¼ cup red pepper, chopped
1 garlic clove, minced
   Pinch of cumin
2 tablespoons no-salt-added chicken broth or 1-2-3 Chicken Broth
   (page 222)
2 eggs, lightly beaten

In a nonstick skillet over medium heat, sauté spinach, red pepper, garlic, and cumin in broth. Pour eggs over spinach and pepper mixture. Reduce heat to low, cover, and cook until eggs are set.

Variation:
For phase 3: top with 1 tablespoon freshly grated Parmesan cheese.

ALL PHASES; SERVES 1

Zesty Mushroom and Asparagus Open Omelet

This is an old standby that I have modified for Fat Flush. The dried mustard gives this dish just the kick it needs.

4   eggs
½   cup steamed asparagus, chopped and drained
½   cup mushrooms, sliced
1   teaspoon purified water
½   teaspoon dried mustard
½   tablespoon fresh parsley, finely minced
½   teaspoon onion powder

Beat eggs in a bowl and stir in remaining ingredients. Pour the egg mixture into a preheated, nonstick skillet and cook over medium heat. As mixture sets, lift up the edges and tilt skillet, so that the uncooked egg flows underneath and sets. When underside is set (about 2 minutes), turn over with a spatula. Cook until bottom is set and turns golden brown. Serve immediately.

Variation:
For phase 3: top with 2 tablespoons of freshly grated Parmesan or Romano cheese.

ALL PHASES; SERVES 2

On-the-Go Omelet

No time to cook? Let the microwave do the work and you're out the door in no time at all.

2   eggs, lightly beaten
1   tomato, chopped
1   scallion, chopped
2   mushrooms, chopped
1   tablespoon parsley, fresh, chopped

Combine all ingredients in a microwavable bowl. Microwave, covered with a paper towel for 1¹/₂ minutes on high, stirring once halfway through the cooking.

Variation:

For phase 3: top with 1 tablespoon of freshly grated Parmesan cheese.

ALL PHASES; SERVES 1

Sprouted Egg Cup

The Ezekiel 4:9 sprouted, whole-grain bread is what makes this breakfast dish so unusual. That, and the dash of fiery cayenne!

1   slice sprouted, whole-grain bread
1   egg
1   teaspoon purified water
1   tablespoon scallions, diced
1   mushroom, finely chopped
    Dash of cayenne

Preheat oven to 350°F. Remove crust from bread and press the remaining bread into a nonstick muffin tin to form a cup. Bake until lightly toasted. Scramble egg with water, scallion, mushroom, and dash of cayenne. Pour into bread cup. Bake until set, about 20–25 minutes. For extra flavor, serve with Fat Flush Catsup (page 206).

PHASES 2 AND 3; SERVES 1

Pico de Gallo Eggs

Here's a sassy breakfast from south of the border, originally created by Claudia Krevat. Also featured on page 208, Pico de Gallo Sauce serves as a condiment in this recipe.

1   cup Pico de Gallo sauce
4   eggs

Warm Pico de Gallo Sauce in a large skillet. When the sauce begins to simmer, add the eggs, and scramble until done. Transfer onto plates. Top each with additional sauce if desired.

Pico de Gallo Sauce

1½ pounds fresh tomatoes, seeded and finely chopped
1   large red onion, finely chopped
2   jalapeños, seeded and minced (optional)
¼   cup fresh cilantro
3   tablespoons fresh lime juice
4   tablespoons no-salt-added chicken broth or 1-2-3 Chicken Broth (page 222)

In a small bowl, mix all ingredients until well blended. Cover and let sit for at least 1 hour before serving.

ALL PHASES; SERVES 2

Goddess Frittata

The nutmeg with the spinach is a delicate touch you will enjoy.

6   eggs, beaten
½   cup nonfat or low-fat cottage cheese
1½ cups fresh or frozen chopped spinach, well drained and patted dry
2   scallions, minced
½   teaspoon basil
¼   teaspoon nutmeg
1   tablespoon butter

Preheat oven to 350°F. Combine eggs, cottage cheese, spinach, scallions, and seasonings. Melt butter in a large ovenproof skillet and add egg mixture. Cook over medium heat for 3 minutes. Place in oven. Bake for another 10 minutes or until set.

PHASE 3; SERVES 4

Laced Artichoke Egg Bake

I like to serve this dish for company. Everyone is always surprised that something so tasty is so very Fat Flush friendly.

2   tablespoons butter
2   tablespoons scallions, chopped
1   tablespoon fresh parsley, chopped
2   teaspoons fresh basil, chopped
8   artichoke hearts, quartered, rinsed, and dried
4   large eggs
4   tablespoons grated Parmesan cheese

Preheat oven to 400°F. Rub butter onto bottom and sides of four ramekins. Sprinkle each with the scallions and herbs. Place 2 artichoke hearts in each dish. Crack 1 egg into each dish. Sprinkle with cheese and bake for about 9 minutes or until eggs set.

PHASE 3; SERVES 2 (TWO RAMEKINS EACH)

Eggs Tex-Mex

So easy, so fast, so good.

2   eggs
1   egg white
    Cayenne to taste
1   ounce Monterey Jack cheese, grated

Whisk eggs and cayenne. Cook in medium skillet over medium heat. Add
  cheese and serve.

Variations:

Experiment with various herb and spice combos:

- For an Asian flavor, mix in a pinch of ginger, coriander, and cayenne.

- For an Indian flavor, mix in a pinch of cumin, turmeric, and coriander.

- For a Greek flavor, mix in a squeeze of lemon and a pinch of oregano.

- For a French flavor, add a drop of white wine, a pinch of tarragon, and
  1 crushed garlic clove.

PHASE 3; SERVES 1

Tofu Scrambler

Perfect for vegetarian Fat Flushers, the turmeric gives this dish the traditional color of real scrambled eggs.

3   tablespoons of 1-2-3 Vegetable Broth (page 221)
½   cup mushrooms
3   tablespoons scallions, chopped
½   garlic clove, minced
1   tablespoon chives, chopped
1   pound soft tofu, drained, rinsed, and squeezed until lightly crumbled
    Pinch of turmeric
2   tablespoons fresh parsley, chopped, for garnish

In a large skillet over medium heat, sauté the mushrooms, scallions, garlic, and chives in the broth until tender. Add in the tofu and turmeric, then scramble until tofu resembles scrambled eggs, about 3 minutes. Garnish with parsley and serve while hot.

ALL PHASES; SERVES 4

Fat Flush Quiche

This is most filling for breakfast, but it serves up nicely as a light lunch or even a snack.

1   slice sprouted, whole-grain bread
1   egg
1   teaspoon purified water
½   ounce Swiss cheese, grated
1   tablespoon onion, diced
1   tablespoon chopped spinach, patted dry and packed
    Dash of cayenne

Preheat oven to 350°F. Remove crust from bread and press remaining bread into a nonstick muffin tin to form a cup. Bake until lightly toasted. Scramble egg with water, cheese, onion, spinach, and cayenne. Pour into bread cup. Bake until set, about 25 minutes.

PHASE 3; SERVES 1

BREAD AND CEREAL

Overnight Oatmeal

This is a great way to cook oatmeal—or brown rice—for those wintry, cold mornings. Cooking on low heat or in a cold oven at 200°F overnight retains optimum mineral values since minerals are easily destroyed at high temperatures.

1   cup steel-cut oats
5   cups purified water, boiled

Combine oats and water in a small Crock-Pot or slow cooker on low heat. Cover and cook on low heat overnight or until done.

Enjoy in the morning!

Variations:

- Add 1 tablespoon of flaxseed oil to the oatmeal after cooking and right before serving or how about a tablespoon or two of Flaxy Butter Spread (page 216)?

- *For phase 3 Special Occasion:* add a spoonful of mixed dried fruits like dates, figs, and apricots. Or sweeten instead with a tablespoon of date sugar or honey.

PHASE 3; SERVES 1

Fat Flush French Toast with Quick Cran-Raspberry Sauce

Serve with Quick Cran-Raspberry Sauce (page 211) for a taste treat that the kids will appreciate, too.

2   slices sprouted, whole-grain bread
2   eggs
1   tablespoon purified water
½   teaspoon cinnamon
¼   teaspoon Stevia Plus
     Quick Cran-Raspberry Sauce

Preheat a nonstick skillet over medium heat. Whisk together eggs, water, cinnamon, and Stevia Plus. Dip each slice of bread in egg mixture until completely coated. Cook over medium heat, about 3 minutes per side.

Variation:
Try the Flaxy Syrup (page 218) instead of the Quick Cran-Raspberry Sauce.

PHASE 3; SERVES 1–2

6 Lunch or Dinner Entrées

Quick and easy but oh so tasty and wholesome. That's the theme for most of the lunch and dinner entrées in this chapter. I have included packable or work-friendly lunches for the working gals and guys out there, such as Stuffed Tomatoes and Lightly Spiced Chicken Wraps as well as quick-fix entrées (who said that egg dishes like the Artichoke Frittata are just for breakfast), main-course salads, casseroles, and one-dish skillet meals that provide comfort food with a bit of flair—the Fat Flush way.

You may be surprised to see that there are many entrées in addition to chicken. In fact, I introduce quite a few entrées made with beef and lamb (including the Warm Thai Lamb Salad and Lamb Salad with Mint). This is not by accident. These protein-rich foods are some of our best sources of both zinc and L-Carnitine—two important nutrients that are lacking in most diets and essential for healing, hormonal balance, and fat burning.

You will also find that onions, leeks, scallions (or green onions), and garlic figure prominently in the entrée section. The onion family is a rich source of sulfur-based compounds and antioxidants, which are cleansing for the liver, anti-inflammatory, and helpful in bringing cholesterol levels down. Garlic, that lovely "stinking rose," contains similar sulfur-based compounds and are believed to contain potent antibiotic, antifungal, and antiparasitic properties.

I know you will enjoy the easy seafood offerings and the kabobs in this section. All of these are designed to provide you with some delicious main courses that take minimal time in the oven, on the grill, or in the skillet.

Fat Flush Secret Tip: **For Phase 3 special occasions you can make any chicken, fish, or lamb dish unique by using a nut crust! In one small bowl, combine 3 or more tablespoons of ground flaxseeds seasoned with your favorite herbs. In another bowl combine ¼ cup Dijon mustard with 2 tablespoons honey. And in a third bowl place ½ cup finely chopped toasted pumpkin seeds, pecans, walnuts, pine nuts, or pistachios. Dip each breast, filet, or chop in the flaxseed mixture, then the honey mustard, and finally the nut mixture to coat. Cook over medium-low heat in a nonstick skillet until cooked through.**

EASY-PACKED LUNCHES

QUICK-FIX ENTRÉES

MAIN DISH SALADS, CASSEROLES, AND ONE-DISH SKILLET MEALS

FISH AND SEAFOOD

EASY-PACKED LUNCHES

Stuffed Tomato with Tuna Salad

This is a great, easy way to bring your lunch to work. Tomatoes, in all forms, are a big Fat Flush favorite because they are a so high in lycopene, the antioxidant found to be protective in prostate and even breast health. The turmeric is delightfully aromatic and therapeutically supports liver function and acts as an anti-inflammatory. Serve with leafy greens and a drizzle of lemon juice.

1   6-ounce canned tuna in water, rinsed and drained
1   tablespoon flaxseed oil
1/4 cup celery, finely chopped
2   tablespoons onion, finely minced
1/2 teaspoon turmeric
1   medium tomato

Mix tuna, flaxseed oil, celery, onion, and turmeric together. Cut off top of tomato about 1/4 of the way down and save top. Scoop out pulp, drain, and stuff with tuna salad. Replace the top of the tomato.

Variations:
- Replace the tuna with salmon, sardines, or mackerel.
- Replace the tomato with a red pepper with the top removed and seeded.
- *For phase 3:* substitute 1/2 an avocado for the tomato. Drizzle with fresh lemon or lime juice and add salt to taste.
- *For phase 3:* how about a couple of tablespoons of chopped walnuts for crunch?

ALL PHASES; SERVES 1

Stuffed Tomato with Deviled Egg Salad

An interesting alternative to our tuna salad, this calls for eggs instead. The mustard gives this egg salad its bite. A side of fresh or lightly steamed spinach is a good accompaniment with just about any of our Fat Flush dressings.

2   eggs, hard-boiled
1/2   tablespoon flaxseed oil
1/2   teaspoon apple cider vinegar
1/4   teaspoon dried mustard
1/2   teaspoon scallions, finely minced
1/4   teaspoon garlic powder
   Pinch of cayenne (optional)
1   medium tomato

Mash eggs. Mix in oil, vinegar, mustard, scallions, garlic, and cayenne. Cut off top of tomato about 1/4 of the way down and save top. Scoop out pulp, drain, and stuff with egg salad. Replace the top of the tomato.

Variations:
- Replace the tomato with a red pepper with the top removed and seeded.
- *For phase 3:* substitute 1/2 an avocado for the tomato. Drizzle with fresh lime or lemon juice and add salt to taste.
- *For phase 3:* a tablespoon of roasted sunflower seeds adds crunch.

ALL PHASES; SERVES 1

Creamy Lemon-Lime Crab Salad

A quickie all-in-one lunch, sweet crab meat is delectable with Creamy Lemon-Lime Yogurt Dressing (page 192). Please note that for those following the Fat Flushing Food Combination rules for phase 3, I consider yogurt (if it is made from whole milk and not nonfat) a dairy fat similar to butter, cream, and sour cream, and so yogurt combines with other protein foods.

1   pound crab, cooked and flaked
3   tablespoons lime juice
½   cup celery, chopped
1¼ cups Creamy Lemon-Lime Yogurt Dressing
4   cups mixed salad greens, shredded
2   tablespoons scallions, finely chopped

Combine all ingredients, except the scallions, in a salad bowl. Mix well and serve. Garnish with scallions.

PHASE 3; SERVES 4

QUICK-FIX ENTRÉES

Artichoke Frittata

This is an easy-to-cook entrée when you don't feel like having heavy proteins at night or at lunch, for that matter. Artichokes contain silymarin—an antioxidant known to help protect the liver from toxic substances.

2   small leeks, sliced, white part only
1   garlic clove, minced
2   scallions, sliced
¼   cup 1-2-3 Vegetable Broth (page 221)
4   eggs, lightly beaten
    Dried dill to taste
2   tablespoons water
1   3½-ounce can artichoke hearts, rinsed and sliced
6   black olives, pitted and minced
2   tablespoons cilantro, chopped
1   teaspoon fresh lemon juice

In a medium, nonstick skillet, sauté leeks, garlic, scallions, and broth until leeks are soft. Spread evenly over the bottom of the skillet. Mix dill and water with eggs and pour into the skillet. Arrange the artichoke slices and olives on top of the egg mixture. Sprinkle with cilantro and cook over low heat until egg mixture is set, about 8 minutes, shaking skillet occasionally. Cover the skillet handle and place under broiler until lightly brown, about 2 minutes. Cut into wedges and drizzle with lemon juice.

Variations:
- A bit of Homemade Salsa (page 207) may be used as a topping.
- *For phase 3:* add salt to taste.

ALL PHASES; SERVES 2

Eggplant Bake

When time is at a premium and you are in the mood for a light meatless supper, this eggplant-based dish works well. Eggplants provide a fleshy, meaty texture which make them a vegetarian favorite and are a decent source of potassium. Serve with Caramelized Onions (page 148).

2   medium eggplants
2   medium onions, chopped
8   garlic cloves, minced
4   tablespoons no-salt-added chicken broth
1   teaspoon ground turmeric
1   teaspoon ground cumin
4   Roma tomatoes, chopped
2   tablespoons fresh cilantro or parsley, chopped
4   eggs, beaten

Preheat oven to 400°F. In oven, roast eggplant whole on nonstick baking sheet until brown on the outside and soft on the inside, testing with a fork, for about 30 minutes or until done. Cool, peel, and mash the pulp. In a large, nonstick skillet or wok, sauté the onions and garlic in the broth until soft, about 20 minutes. Stir in mashed eggplant, add turmeric and cumin, and sauté for another 2 minutes. Add tomatoes and cook for 5 minutes. Add the cilantro or parsley and the eggs, stirring until cooked through and eggs set.

Serve piping hot.

Variation:

For phase 3: add salt to taste.

ALL PHASES; SERVES 2

MAIN DISH SALADS, CASSEROLES, AND ONE-DISH SKILLET MEALS

Warm Thai Lamb Salad

The Thai spices provide an exotic accompaniment to this dish, and they take the edge off the distinctive lamb flavor. Serve on a bed of steamed greens with Garlicky Avocado Dressing (page 194).

1   pound (16 ounces) shoulder lamb chops, deboned
1   teaspoon ground coriander
1/2 teaspoon ground cumin
1/2 teaspoon ground ginger
1/4 teaspoon ground anise
1   carrot, peeled and thinly sliced in strips
1   red pepper, seeded and sliced thinly
1   zucchini, thinly sliced in strips
1   bunch scallions
1   4-ounce can water chestnuts, drained, rinsed, and sliced
1/2 cucumber, thinly sliced in strips
1   cup bean sprouts
1½ cups Garlicky Avocado Dressing
     Salt to taste

Preheat oven to 400°F. Rub lamb with spices. Place lamb in a nonstick roasting pan and roast for about 15–20 minutes until cooked through. Remove from pan, leaving juices from the lamb in the pan, set aside, and let cool.

Place carrot, red pepper, zucchini, scallions, and water chestnuts in the roasting pan and stir into the juices. Roast the vegetables for 2–3 minutes to soften. Remove from pan and place into a large bowl and cool. Add cucumber and bean sprouts to the roasted veggie mixture and toss.

Slice the lamb into thin strips and combine with the veggie mixture. Spoon Garlicy Avocado Dressing over the lamb-veggie mixture, season, and serve at room temperature.

PHASE 3; SERVES 4

Lamb Salad with Mint

This dish is a natural with Minty Sesame Dressing (page 197) and provides a refreshing Middle Eastern flavor.

1 pound lean lamb roast, cooked and thinly sliced
2 cups cauliflower florets, steamed
¼ cup Minty Sesame Dressing
4 cups mixed salad greens, shredded
    Sprigs of mint

Combine the lamb and cauliflower in a large serving bowl. Add the dressing, cover, and marinate for at least 1 hour in the fridge. Take out of the fridge and toss in shredded salad greens. Garnish with sprigs of mint.

Variation:

Insert slivers of garlic into the lamb roast and rub with dried rosemary before cooking.

PHASE 3; SERVES 4

Mexican Salad

The cumin, cayenne, and garlic give this all-in-one salad a south of the border flair.

1   pound flank steak, thinly sliced
2   tablespoons 1-2-3 Beef Broth (page 223)
1   onion, chopped
4   garlic cloves, minced
2   teaspoons ground cumin
1   teaspoon cayenne
¼   cup no-salt-added tomato sauce
2   tablespoons tomato paste
1   tablespoon apple cider vinegar
    Salt to taste
8   cups leafy greens (romaine, spinach, mixed lettuces)
3   scallions, sliced
2   tomatoes, chopped
¼   cup black olives
    Baked tortilla chips or blue corn chips

In a nonstick skillet, brown flank steak over medium heat. Cook until steak is almost cooked through. Add two tablespoons of broth. Add onion and garlic and cook for 2 minutes. Add cumin, cayenne, tomato sauce, tomato paste, vinegar, and salt. Heat until lightly bubbly, reduce heat, and simmer for 10–15 minutes. Place 2 cups of greens per serving on a plate. Top with beef mixture, scallions, tomatoes, and olives. Serve with a side of chips.

Variation:

For phases 1 and 2: omit the salt and chips.

PHASE 3; SERVES 4

Baked Chicken and Artichoke Casserole

This is a comforting one-dish meal that's sure to please.

2   5-ounce chicken breasts, boneless and skinless
1   cup 1-2-3 Chicken Broth (page 222)
½   medium red onion, diced
1   red bell pepper, chopped
1   8-ounce can artichoke hearts, rinsed, and drained
4   garlic cloves, minced
6   black olives, chopped
    Juice of 1 lemon
1   8-ounce can no-salt-added tomato sauce
    Handful of fresh cilantro, chopped

Preheat oven to 350°F. In a medium pot, place chicken breasts and broth and simmer. Poach chicken until tender. When cooked, shred chicken into bite-sized pieces. Place chicken, onion, red bell pepper, artichoke hearts, garlic, olives, and lemon juice in a medium casserole dish and mix well. Cover and bake in oven for 45 minutes. Stir tomato sauce into the casserole and return to oven for 20 minutes uncovered. Mix in cilantro and serve.

Variations:
- *For phases 2 and 3:* try replacing the cilantro with a tablespoon of fresh basil for a Mediterranean feel.
- *For phase 3:* stir in 1 tablespoon of sherry during the last 10 minutes of cooking.

ALL PHASES; SERVES 2

Chicken Stir-Fry with a Touch of Turmeric

A key ingredient in Indian dishes, turmeric is a wonderful Fat Flush seasoning because it helps to tone the liver, is a blood sugar regulator, and is especially high in beta-carotene, a nutrient known to support skin health. Its musky warm aroma is very inviting. Serve with Tangy Pickled Cauliflower (page 149).

¼ cup no-salt-added chicken broth or 1-2-3 Chicken Broth (page 222)
1 medium onion, cut into ½-inch slices
1 cup mushrooms, sliced
1 pound chicken breast, boned, skinned, and cut into strips
½ cup water chestnuts
2 cups broccoli florets
2 cups cauliflower florets
1 teaspoon ground turmeric
1 teaspoon ground cumin

In a large, nonstick skillet, heat broth over medium heat. Add onion and cook until soft, about 3–5 minutes. Add mushrooms and cook until soft, about another 1 minute. Add chicken and cook an additional 5 minutes. Finally, add water chestnuts, broccoli, cauliflower, and spices. Cook until tender, another 6 minutes. Ready to serve.

Variations:
- You may use turkey instead of the chicken.
- *For phase 3:* add ⅛ teaspoon ground saffron over the top with a squeeze of lime.

ALL PHASES; SERVES 4

Hearty Turkey Squash Stew with Apricots

The apricots in this dish provide a kind of lemony bite that meshes nicely with the exotic flavors of the coriander, cumin, cloves, and anise. Apricots are a good source of iron as well as other trace minerals, which makes them a lovely nutritional adjunct to any special occasion. The addition of the apricots to this dish is not for those strictly following the Fat Flushing Food Combination rules.

1	teaspoon ground coriander
1	teaspoon ground cumin
	Dash of ground cloves
	Dash of ground anise
1/4	teaspoon cayenne
	Salt to taste
1	pound turkey breast, boned, skinned, and cut into 1-inch pieces
1/4	plus 1 cup 1-2-3 Chicken Broth (page 222), divided
1/2	onion, halved and thinly sliced
1	pound butternut squash, cut into 1-inch cubes
4	ounces apricots, dried, unsulfured
1	cup purified water
2	tablespoons scallions, finely chopped

In a medium bowl, place coriander, cumin, cloves, anise, cayenne, salt, and turkey and toss to coat. In a large pot over medium heat, heat 1/4 cup broth. Add turkey and cook for 4–5 minutes. Add onion, squash, apricots, and remaining 1 cup of broth. Bring mixture to a boil, adding water as needed. Reduce heat to low, cover, and simmer until squash is tender. Serve hot with a sprinkle of scallions as garnish.

PHASE 3 SPECIAL OCCASION; SERVES 4

Slow-Cooker Beef Stew

No time to fuss when you come from work? Then pop this into your slow cooker or Crock-Pot before you leave for work in the morning, and you will have a comforting stew as your reward. Slow cooking over low heat makes the stew meat as tender as butter (or should I say flaxseed oil?).

1½ pounds stew meat, lean, and trimmed of all visible fat, cut into chunks

4   Roma tomatoes, cut into chunks

2   scallions, thinly sliced

1   teaspoon Fat Flush Curry Seasoning (page 204)

1   teaspoon cayenne

1   small head cauliflower, cut into florets

1   small head broccoli, cut into florets

1   carrot, grated

1   cup purified water

Mix all ingredients in a 3½ quart or larger slow cooker. Cover and cook on low for 6 to 8 hours until beef is cooked through and vegetables are tender.

Variations:
- *For phase 2:* add 1 small sweet potato.
- *For phase 3:* replace 1 cup of water with 1 cup of sherry.

ALL PHASES; SERVES 4

Ultimate Beef Brisket with Vegetables and Gravy

When you've got time on the weekends, this stew will keep you satisfied. It is also a good slow cooker meal that will greet and meet you after work.

1	3-pound beef brisket, trimmed
2	cups 1-2-3 Beef Broth (page 223)
1	large onion stuck with 3 whole cloves
3	large carrots, cut into chunks
4	celery stalks with leaves, cut into 1-inch pieces
1	bay leaf
3	garlic cloves, minced
1/2	cup cauliflower florets
3	small carrots, cut into chunks
4	small whole onions, peeled
1/2	small head of cabbage, quartered
1/2	teaspoon cayenne

In a large kettle, sear beef brisket over medium heat until browned. Pour off fat.

Add broth, onion, large carrot, celery, bay leaf, and garlic. Cover, bring to a boil, reduce heat, and simmer 1 1/2 hours. Remove vegetables and bay leaf—reserve for gravy. Add remaining vegetables in order given: cauliflower, small carrots, and onions. Sprinkle cabbage with cayenne, then add to pot. Cover and simmer an additional 1 1/2 hours or until meat is tender and vegetables are cooked but not soggy. Transfer to serving platter.

Gravy

Mash vegetables and bay leaf set aside earlier into meat broth from kettle. Bring to a boil and reduce to desired consistency. Remove bay leaf. To serve, slice cooked brisket in 1-inch slices and surround with vegetables. Spoon gravy over brisket.

Variation:
For phase 2 and 3: add 1 large sweet potato, cut into chunks.

ALL PHASES; SERVES 4

Fat Flush Shepherd's Pie

Here's a delicious classic that works well with Kari's Marvelously Mashed Cauliflower (page 143).

1	pound lean ground beef
1	medium onion, chopped
4	garlic cloves, minced
1	green pepper, chopped
8	ounces mushrooms, sliced
1	teaspoon cayenne
1/2	teaspoon onion powder
1/2	teaspoon garlic powder
2	small carrots, grated
12	black olives, pitted and chopped
	Handful of fresh cilantro, chopped
1	8-ounce can no-salt-added tomato sauce
1	14 1/2-ounce can no-salt-added diced tomato
2	cups mashed cauliflower, as prepared in Kari's Marvelously Mashed Cauliflower

Preheat oven to 350°F. In a large, nonstick skillet, brown ground beef, onion, and garlic. When beef is nearly done, add green pepper, mushrooms, cayenne, onion powder, and garlic powder. When beef is no longer pink, transfer to a large casserole dish. Add carrots, olives, cilantro, tomato sauce, and diced tomatoes to casserole dish and mix well. Spread mashed cauliflower over the top. Bake in oven for 30 minutes. Place under broiler for 3 minutes or until browned on top.

Variations:

- Ground turkey may be used instead of beef.
- *For phase 3:* add 1/2 teaspoon of salt to the casserole mixture before baking.

ALL PHASES; SERVES 4

Stuffed Onion Casserole

This is an unusual casserole that serves up nicely with Hearty Barbecue Sauce (page 210). The secret here is to blanch the onions before filling them so they will hold up better when they are cooking.

4   extra large onions, peeled, cut in half crosswise, with centers
    removed and three layers of onions still intact
1   green pepper, chopped
1   pound lean ground beef
1   egg, beaten
1   teaspoon garlic powder
    Handful of fresh cilantro, chopped
1   cup Hearty Barbecue Sauce

Preheat oven to 350°F. Blanch onion halves in hot water and set aside. Chop the onion centers to make 3/4 cup. Combine chopped onion, green pepper, ground beef, egg, garlic powder, cilantro, and 1/2 cup of the Hearty Barbecue Sauce. Mix well and make four large meatballs. Stuff meatballs into the four onion halves and place the top half of the onions over the meatballs, making sure there is a gap between the top and bottom of the onion. Place stuffed onions in a shallow baking pan and bake for 50–60 minutes. Baste with remaining Hearty Barbecue Sauce during the last 15 minutes of cooking.

Variation:
Ground turkey may be used instead of beef.

ALL PHASES; SERVES 4

Hearty Mushroom Chili

You won't be missing the beans with this chili. The mushrooms are a great bean substitute and provide lots of healthy B vitamins, which are so good for the nervous system and the skin. Accompany with a nice leafy green salad and a Fat Flush dressing of your choice.

1	pound lean ground beef
1	cup onions, chopped
4	garlic cloves, minced
1	green pepper, chopped
1	pound mushrooms, sliced
12	black olives, chopped
1	28-ounce can no-salt-added tomato puree
2	14½-ounce cans no-salt-added diced tomatoes
1	tablespoon ground fennel
1	teaspoon ground cumin
1	teaspoon garlic powder
1	teaspoon onion powder
	Cayenne to taste
	Juice of 1 lime
	Fresh cilantro for garnish

In a large pot over medium heat, place the beef, onions, and garlic and brown until beef is nearly done. Add green pepper and mushrooms and cook until beef is no longer pink. Stir in remaining ingredients except cilantro. Bring to a boil, reduce heat, and simmer for at least 1 hour. Garnish with cilantro just before serving. Freezes well.

Variation:
For phase 3: add ½ teaspoon of salt to the seasonings.

ALL PHASES; SERVES 4

Rosemary Lamb Casserole

Lamb is one of my personal favorite Fat Flushing foods because it is a great source of the amino acidlike substance L-Carnitine, which is a valuable weight-loss nutrient and speeds up the rate at which the body metabolizes fat in the liver. If you can buy New Zealand lamb, all the better; New Zealand lamb is grass-fed. Lightly steamed asparagus or green beans with a drizzle of flaxseed oil or a touch of sesame oil go nicely with this lamb dish.

1   pound lean lamb, trimmed and cut into cubes
1   onion, chopped
2   garlic cloves, minced
1   green pepper, chopped
1   red pepper, chopped
1   teaspoon dried rosemary
1¼ cup 1-2-3 Beef Broth (page 223)
2   cups tomatoes, chopped
2   jalapeños, seeded and minced (optional)
     Salt to taste
2   scallions, chopped

Preheat oven to 300°F. In a large, nonstick skillet over medium heat, place lamb, onion, garlic, peppers, and rosemary. Cook until meat is browned. Add broth, tomatoes, jalapeños, and salt to skillet and boil for 1 minute. Transfer to covered casserole and cook in the oven for 1½ hours or until meat is tender. Top with scallions and serve.

Variation:

For special occasion: 2 tablespoons of burgundy may be added to the casserole during the last 30 minutes of cooking.

PHASE 3; SERVES 4

Tofu-Veggie Stir-Sauté

Try this vegetarian dish as a change from meat.

¼   cup no-salt-added vegetable broth or 1-2-3 Vegetable Broth
     (page 221)
2   garlic cloves, minced
2   cups broccoli florets
1   red pepper, cut into 1-inch squares
1   cup asparagus, cut into 1-inch lengths
1   cup zucchini, halved and cut into ½-inch slices
1   carrot, thinly sliced
1   leek, cut into ¼-inch slices
1   tomato, cut into small cubes
1   pound firm tofu, washed, drained, and cut into 1-inch cubes

In a large, nonstick skillet, heat broth over medium heat. Add garlic and sauté for 1 minute. Add broccoli, red pepper, asparagus, zucchini, and carrot and stir-sauté until crisp-tender. Add leek and tomato and stir-sauté for 2 minutes. Add tofu and stir sauté until tofu is heated through.

Variation:

For phase 3: add salt to season or 2 tablespoons tamari.

ALL PHASES; SERVES 4

FISH AND SEAFOOD

Easy Broiled Salmon

Salmon is a Fat Flush favorite fish, and for good reason. It is high in metabolism revving omega-3s and tasty as well. Serve with steamed broccoli (page 128) and drizzle with flaxseed oil and a squeeze of lemon.

3   tablespoons lemon juice
2   tablespoons fresh parsley, chopped
2   tablespoons cilantro, chopped
2   garlic cloves, minced
2   teaspoons ground cumin
1/4 teaspoon cayenne
4   5-ounce salmon fillets

Combine lemon juice, parsley, cilantro, garlic, cumin, and cayenne ingredients in a medium bowl. Add the fillets and rub the mixture in until fillets are well coated on both sides. Chill and marinate for at least 1 hour. Preheat broiler. Place fish in a nonstick broiling pan under broiler and cook for about 4 minutes on each side or until salmon is opaque in the center. Serve immediately.

Variations:
- *For phase 3:* add 4 tablespoons of white wine to the marinade and sprinkle 1 tablespoon of slivered almonds on top of fish fillet before serving.
- *For phase 3:* accompany with 1/2 cup of brown rice.

ALL PHASES; SERVES 4

Simply Baked Fish

Fat Flushers find this recipe easy and fast. It lends itself beautifully to any white fish. Serve with Dilly Okra (page 138).

1   5-ounce fish fillet (halibut, cod, grouper, flounder)
4   tablespoons lemon juice
1   clove garlic, minced
1   tablespoon fresh parsley, chopped
1   teaspoon gingerroot, grated
    Lemon wedges for garnish

Preheat oven to 350°F. Place all ingredients in a bowl, mix well, making sure fillets are evenly coated with spices. Let stand for 15 minutes. Place fish in a shallow, nonstick pan and bake for about 12 minutes or until the fish is flaky. Baste occasionally with the marinade. Garnish with a lemon wedge. Serve immediately.

Variations:
- *For phase 2:* substitute oregano or rosemary for the gingerroot.
- *For phase 3:* substitute thyme for the gingerroot and add a pinch of salt to taste.

ALL PHASES; SERVES 1

Gingerly Grilled Salmon

Ginger goes well with any fish, but it has a special affinity for salmon.

4   tablespoons 1-2-3 Vegetable Broth (page 221)
1   bay leaf, finely chopped
5   garlic cloves, minced
4   5-ounce salmon fillets
1   tablespoon apple cider vinegar
⅛   teaspoon ground ginger
10   black olives, chopped
1   tomato, chopped
½   red onion, sliced

Place 2 tablespoons of the broth plus the bay leaf and garlic in a small
bowl. In a glass baking dish, coat fish with herb mixture and arrange
coated fish in a single layer in the dish. Cover and refrigerate for at
least 2 hours or overnight. Whisk remaining broth, vinegar, and ginger in a medium bowl. Add olives, tomato and red onion. Set aside.
Preheat broiler. Grill or broil salmon for about 9 minutes or until
salmon is opaque in the center. Transfer to serving plates and top with
olives, tomato, and onion.

ALL PHASES; SERVES 4

Salmon Cakes

These cakes are certainly savory just the way they are. However, when you move on to phase 3, try them with Gingered Asparagus (page 151) and a tablespoon or two of Minty Dill Pesto (page 213) for a special flavor and natural digestive aid treat.

8   ounces cooked salmon fillet, skinned
¼   cup scallions, finely chopped
2   teaspoons fresh dill
2   garlic cloves, minced
     Splash of fresh lemon juice
1   egg, beaten

Preheat oven to 350°F. Place salmon in a large bowl and separate with a fork. Mix in scallions, dill, garlic, lemon juice, and egg. Shape mixture into two patties, about 3/4 inch thick. Place patties in nonstick baking dish or nonstick baking sheet in oven. Bake in oven for about 15 minutes or until golden brown and cooked through.

Variation:

For phase 2 and 3: add ¼ cup of Ezekiel 4:9 bread crumbs to the ingredients.

ALL PHASES; SERVES 2

Seafood Kebabs

Seafood Kebabs are Fat Flush favorites for parties and cookouts. This recipe calls for 8 skewers.

1   pound white fish (cod, sole, or flounder), cut into 1-inch cubes
2   lemons, juiced
1   tablespoon no-salt-added vegetable broth or 1-2-3 Vegetable
    Broth (page 221)
3   tablespoons fresh parsley, chopped
1   teaspoon fresh ginger, grated, or dash of dried ginger
2   garlic cloves, minced
6   baby zucchinis each cut into four chunks
16 button mushrooms
8   cherry tomatoes

In a large bowl, marinate the fish with lemon juice, broth, parsley, ginger, and garlic, cover, and refrigerate for 1 hour, turning fish over every 20 minutes. Preheat broiler for 5 minutes on high. Remove fish from marinade. Using skewers, thread the fish, zucchinis, mushrooms, and tomatoes alternately. Grill/broil for about 10 minutes, turning occasionally, until fish is cooked through.

Variation:
For phase 3: you may add a splash of dry vermouth to the marinade.

ALL PHASES; SERVES 4

Asian Scallops

*The fragrant spices of this dish marry well with Mashed Celery Root (page 144)
and will transport you to far away, exotic places.*

¼ cup 1-2-3 Vegetable Broth (page 221)
1   pound scallops, rinsed and dried
1   tablespoon shallots, finely minced
1   teaspoon ground coriander
1   teaspoon dried fennel
¼ teaspoon ground cumin
⅛ teaspoon turmeric
    Lemon slices

In a large, nonstick skillet, heat the broth over high heat. Add the scallops
to the skillet, stirring lightly with a wooden spoon and cook for about
1 minute. Add shallots, coriander, fennel, cumin, and turmeric to the
scallops, and cook for about 3 minutes turning scallops until they are
golden or lightly browned. Add a squeeze of lemon juice before
removing from heat. Serve piping hot.

Variation:
For phase 3: add 2 tablespoons of sherry to the skillet.

ALL PHASES; SERVES 4

Marinated Shrimp over Squash

If spaghetti squash is not in season, you can use zucchini or summer squash instead. All these squash are mild tasting and will absorb the flavors of the marinated shrimp quite nicely. Serve with Spiced Vanilla Peaches (page 256) to complement the delicious bouquet of flavors presented in this dish.

4   tomatoes, chopped
5   scallions, chopped
3   garlic cloves, minced
1   tablespoon fresh parsley, chopped
1   tablespoon fresh cilantro, chopped
¼   cup apple cider vinegar
2   teaspoons fresh gingerroot, grated
1   teaspoon cayenne
½   teaspoon dried chives
½   teaspoon onion powder
6   black olives, chopped
     Juice of 2 limes
     Juice of 1 lemon
1   cup 1-2-3 Vegetable Broth (page 221)
8   ounces large shrimps, peeled and deveined
1   medium spaghetti squash, as prepared in Fat Flush Spaghetti with
     Meat Sauce (page 114)

In a large covered bowl, combine tomatoes, scallions, garlic, parsley, cilantro, vinegar, gingerroot, cayenne, chives, onion powder, olives, lime and lemon juice, and vegetable broth and let marinate for 30 minutes in the refrigerator. Place marinade in large saucepan or medium, nonstick skillet and bring to a boil. Reduce heat to simmer, add shrimp, and cook for about 1½ minutes. Turn shrimp for another 1½ minutes until pink and firm. Remove from heat and serve over spaghetti squash.

ALL PHASES; SERVES 2

Shrimp Stuffed Portobello Mushrooms

The shrimp and portobello mushrooms are a meaty combination that provides satiety and satisfaction.

2   celery stalks, chopped
2   scallions, chopped
4   button mushrooms, chopped
2   garlic cloves, chopped
4   tablespoons 1-2-3 Vegetable Broth, divided (page 221)
8   ounces of shrimp, peeled, deveined, and cooked
6   black olives, chopped
1   Roma tomato, chopped
4   tablespoons no-salt-added tomato sauce
    Pinch of cayenne
    Juice of ½ lemon
1   tablespoon fresh cilantro, chopped
6   portobello mushroom caps (approximately 4 inches in diameter),
    with underside brown gills removed

Preheat oven to 400°F. In a nonstick skillet over medium heat, sauté celery, scallions, button mushrooms, and garlic in 2 tablespoons broth for 8 to 10 minutes or until soft, adding more broth as needed. Place sautéed veggies in food processor with cooked shrimp and all remaining ingredients except portobello caps. Pulse processor about 10 times until mixture is finely chopped. Place spoonfuls of mixture on the underside of the portobello mushrooms. Bake on nonstick baking sheet for 30 minutes. Serve immediately.

ALL PHASES; SERVES 2 (3 CAPS APIECE)

Sassy Sole Loaf

Light and airy, this loaf is quite easy to put together, and you can use any fish you wish.

3   eggs, whites and yolks separated
2½ cups sole, cooked and flaked
½   cup Fat Flush Bread Crumbs (page 203)
1   teaspoon cayenne
1   teaspoon garlic powder
1   teaspoon onion powder
1   teaspoon dried dill

Preheat oven to 350°F. Beat the egg yolks until foamy, and the whites until soft peaks form. Combine all the remaining ingredients and add to the egg yolks. Carefully blend in the egg whites. Pour into a nonstick loaf pan and bake for about 40–50 minutes or until done.

Variation:

Experiment with different spices such as ½ teaspoon of dried basil and oregano instead of garlic and onion powders to make this a Sole Loaf Italiano.

PHASES 2 AND 3; SERVES 4

Saucy Cucumber Basil Halibut

Unlike many of the other recipes in which you may use dried herbs for fresh, the basil really needs to be fresh in this fish dish. The pungent taste of fresh basil truly sets off the whole recipe and makes the dish a refreshing entrée for a summery kind of day.

4   5-ounce halibut fillets
    Juice of ½ lemon
1   pound cucumber, skinned and grated
1   cup plain, whole milk yogurt
1½ teaspoons fresh lemon juice
3   teaspoons fresh basil, chopped

Preheat oven to 300°F. Place fillets in a nonstick baking dish or on a nonstick baking sheet. Squeeze the lemon over the top of the fish. Bake, uncovered for about 10 to 15 minutes (depending upon thickness of the fish) or until fish is cooked and flakes easily with a fork. While fish is in the oven, place the cucumber, yogurt, lemon juice, and basil in a large, nonstick skillet to make sauce. Cook over low heat until sauce is hot, making sure that sauce doesn't boil. Serve fish topped with sauce.

Variation:

As an alternative to the fresh basil, 1 teaspoon of dried oregano or dill will give this dish some zip.

PHASE 3; SERVES 4

Crispy Nonfried Fish

Here is the Fat Flush version of fried fish. I served this to my nephews Isaac and Daniel, who are my most honest taste testers. They don't understand what the fuss is all about—it's just fried fish. Serve with Jícama Slaw (page 133).

1   egg, beaten
¼   teaspoon ginger
1   cup Fat Flush bread crumbs (page 203)
½   teaspoon garlic powder
¼   teaspoon cayenne
¼   teaspoon dried mustard
4   5-ounce fish fillets (sole, sea bass, cod)
     Juice of 1 lemon
     Fresh parsley for garnish

Preheat oven to 475°F. In a large bowl, combine the beaten egg and ginger. In another bowl, mix together the bread crumbs, garlic powder, cayenne, and dried mustard. Dip each fillet into the egg mixture, and then coat it with the seasoned bread crumb mixture. Place the fillets on a nonstick cooking sheet. Bake for about 8 minutes or until fish is golden or cooked through. Squeeze lemon juice over the fish. Garnish with parsley, and serve.

Variation:
Use chicken breasts instead of fish.

PHASES 2 AND 3; SERVES 4

POULTRY

Limey Chicken

The coriander imparts a currylike flavor. Coriander is a marvelous spice that is from the seed of the cilantro plant. Serve with Broccoli-Cauliflower Salad (page 132).

Juice of 2 limes
1 garlic clove, minced
½ teaspoon dried ginger
½ teaspoon coriander
4 5-ounce chicken thighs or breasts, skinned
Lemon slices for garnish

Preheat oven to 350°F. In a small bowl, combine lime juice, garlic, ginger, and coriander. Rub mixture onto chicken. Place chicken in nonstick casserole dish or baking pan and cover. Bake about 45 minutes or until tender. Serve hot, garnished with lemon slices.

Variation:
For phase 3: you may add ½ teaspoon of salt to spice mixture.

ALL PHASES; SERVES 4

Turkey and Okra Casserole

This dish is a little more time-consuming than many of the others but is well worth it. Okra is one of my all-time favorite vegetables for Fat Flushers because it is one of the richest vegetable sources of fiber—so good for maintaining regularity, bringing down cholesterol, and stabilizing blood sugar. The okra in this recipe provides 12 grams of fiber—4 grams in each ½ cup. Okra is a decent source of vitamin C, beta-carotene, and the B-complex vitamins.

1   pound ground turkey

3   cups okra, chopped and divided

2   cups green pepper, chopped and divided

2   cups onion, chopped and divided

2   cups eggplant, peeled, diced, and divided

¼   plus ½ cup 1-2-3 Chicken Broth (page 222), divided

1½ teaspoons onion powder

1   teaspoon dried mustard

1   teaspoon garlic powder

½   teaspoon dried dill

1   teaspoon ground cumin

      Cayenne to taste

¼   cup apple cider vinegar

2   14½-ounce cans no-salt-added diced tomatoes

½   cup tomato sauce

Preheat oven to 350°F. In a large, nonstick skillet over medium heat, brown ground turkey until cooked. Transfer turkey to a platter and set aside. Combine 1 cup of okra, 1 cup of green pepper, 1 cup of onion, and 1 cup of eggplant in a food processor, pulsing until very finely chopped. Place ¼ cup broth, finely chopped veggie mixture, and spices and herbs in nonstick skillet and cook over medium heat for about 5 minutes, stirring constantly to prevent sticking and burning until veggies are crisp-tender and lightly browned. Stir in vinegar, remaining broth, and tomatoes and continue cooking for about 20 minutes, stirring until most of liquid evaporates. Add in the remaining okra, green pepper, onion, eggplant, and tomato sauce and cook 10 minutes more. In a large, covered casserole dish, combine cooked turkey and veggie mixture and bake for 20 minutes. Serve.

Variations:

- *For phase 1:* to enhance digestion, try adding 1/2–1 tablespoon of fennel to the spices for a delicate and subtle taste treat and settled stomach.
- *For phase 1:* you might garnish with 4 tablespoons of cilantro.
- *For phase 1:* you could also garnish with 2 tablespoons of fresh parsley and 2 tablespoons of cilantro.
- *For phase 2:* you might wish to add 1/2 tablespoon of dried basil to the spices.
- *For phase 3:* you may add salt to taste before baking the dish in the oven.

ALL PHASES; SERVES 4

Chicken with Dill

This is as easy as can be. I have used this recipe many times when I have come home from work. I put it all together even before I took my coat off. Serve with Fat Flush Ratatouille (page 136).

2   5-ounce chicken breasts, boned, skinned, and halved
3   garlic cloves, minced
½   teaspoon dried dill
¼   cup fresh lemon juice
½   cup 1-2-3 Chicken Broth (page 222)

Preheat oven to 350°F. Rub chicken with garlic. Place in baking dish and
   sprinkle with dill and lemon juice. Pour chicken broth over chicken.
   Bake for 45 minutes or until chicken is cooked through.

ALL PHASES; SERVES 2

Tangy Chicken with Tomatillos

Tomatillos, most commonly used in salsas, have a sweet-and-sour flavor which provides this dish with a most memorable and tangy taste. Kari's Marvelously Mashed Cauliflower (page 143) is an integral component of this taste sensation, which, I predict, will become one of your most requested entrees. Many thanks to Kari Wheaton, who created this recipe for me.

4   5-ounce chicken breasts, skinned, boned, and cubed
1½ teaspoons ground cumin
½   teaspoon cayenne
1   teaspoon garlic powder
¼   cup 1-2-3 Chicken Broth (page 222), divided
1   cup onion, chopped
4   garlic cloves, minced
4   cups tomatillos, chopped
2   cups mashed cauliflower, as prepared in Kari's Marvelously Mashed Cauliflower
2   cups cherry tomatoes, halved
1   cup fresh cilantro, chopped

In a medium bowl, combine chicken breasts, cumin, cayenne, and garlic powder, making sure to evenly coat chicken with spices. In a large, nonstick skillet on medium heat, heat 1/8 cup of the broth, add chicken mixture, and sauté for 5 minutes. Remove from skillet onto a plate and set aside. Heat remaining broth in skillet on medium heat and add onion and garlic cloves, sautéing about 2 minutes until tender. Add tomatillos and sauté for another 2 minutes. Add mashed cauliflower and the chicken mixture back to skillet, cover, and cook for 10 minutes or until chicken is thoroughly cooked. Add tomatoes and cilantro, cover, and cook for 2 minutes and serve.

ALL PHASES; SERVES 4

Lightly Spiced Chicken Wraps

A great lunch for taking to work and is actually easier than it sounds. You can pack the chicken and cabbage mixtures into baggies and microwave these as needed to serve over the Romaine lettuce leaves.

2   5-ounce chicken breasts, skinned, boned, and halved
1   teaspoon ground cumin
½   teaspoon cayenne
½   teaspoon cinnamon
2   teaspoons plus 1 tablespoon fresh ginger, minced
1   tablespoon fresh parsley, chopped
3   garlic cloves, minced and divided
2   tablespoons apple cider vinegar
½   cup no-salt-added chicken broth
⅛   teaspoon Stevia Plus (optional)
1   jalapeño, minced (optional)
3   scallions, sliced
1   medium onion, chopped
1   green pepper, sliced
1   carrot shredded
6   cups Napa cabbage, thinly sliced
1   cup cilantro, chopped
1   tablespoon flaxseed oil
    Juice of 1 lime
    Romaine lettuce leaves

Place chicken breasts in a plastic bag with the cumin, cayenne, cinnamon, 2 teaspoons of ginger, parsley, and 1 clove of garlic. Seal bag and place in fridge. Let spices coat chicken and be absorbed for at least 1 hour or overnight. Preheat oven to 350°F. Remove chicken from bag, place in a nonstick baking dish and bake for about 30 minutes or until cooked through. In a small bowl, make a dressing by combining vinegar, broth, ⅛ teaspoon Stevia Plus, remaining ginger, remaining garlic cloves, and jalapeno. In a large saucepan, combine the dressing with scallions, onion, and green pepper and sauté for 2 to 3 minutes. Add carrot and cabbage and cook for an additional 5 minutes. Remove from heat and toss in cilantro, flaxseed oil, and lime juice. Slice chicken breasts into thin strips and serve on Romaine lettuce leaves with the cabbage mixture.

Variations:

- Use 1/2 pound flank steak instead of chicken.
- Or how about substituting turkey breasts for the chicken?
- *For phase 2:* you might replace the cumin, cayenne, and cinnamon with 2 teaspoons of Chinese 5-spice Powder for an exotic touch.
- *For phase 2:* add 1/2 teaspoon of dried basil to the spices.
- *For phase 3:* try adding a pinch of salt.

ALL PHASES; SERVES 2

Faux Chicken Fried Rice

This is another variation on the cauliflower theme which integrates Kari's Marvelously Mashed Cauliflower (page 143). Cauliflower is not your ordinary starch substitute for mashed potatoes or rice. It is a highly regarded member of the cruciferous family and contains many anticancerous substances. As Mark Twain once said, "Cauliflower is nothing but cabbage with a college education."

1   medium onion, chopped
2   garlic cloves, minced
2   carrots, grated
8   tablespoons of no-salt-added chicken broth, divided
2   stalks celery, chopped
1   can water chestnuts, chopped
2   5-ounce chicken breasts, cooked, skinned, boned, and diced
1   cup mashed cauliflower, cooked as in Kari's Marvelously Mashed
    Cauliflower
2   eggs, beaten
    Juice of 1 lemon

Sauté onion, garlic, and carrots in 4 tablespoons of the chicken broth in a
    nonstick pan until onions are caramelized—about 20 minutes. Add
    celery and water chestnuts and cook for about 5 minutes or until
    crisp-tender. Add remaining broth, chicken, and mashed cauliflower
    and cook through. Add eggs and cook until eggs set, stirring well.
    Add lemon juice and serve.

Variation:
For phase 3: you may add salt to taste.

ALL PHASES; SERVES 2

Roast Turkey with Lemon, Garlic, and Fennel

Turkey is a great staple for the whole week. Turkey slices can be used as quick snacks and placed in the 1-2-3 Chicken Broth (page 222) for turkey soup. The lemon, garlic, and fennel help with digestion to make this bird Fat Flush friendly.

1   5- to 6-pound whole turkey breast
     Zest of 1 lemon
     Juice of 1 lemon
2   garlic cloves, minced
2   teaspoons fennel, ground
3   tablespoons 1-2-3 Chicken Broth (page 222)
2   fresh lemons, halved

Preheat oven to 425°F. In a bowl, mix lemon zest, lemon juice, garlic, fennel, and chicken broth. Rub turkey with herb mixture and place the halved lemons on top. Place turkey in a roasting pan and roast for 20 minutes. Lower the oven to 325°F and roast for another 1³/4 hours, basting with pan drippings. When done, juices from the thickest part of the turkey should run clear. Remove from oven and cool for 20 minutes before carving.

Variations:
- *For phases 2 and 3:* serve with Puréed Sweet Potatoes (page 153).
- *For phase 3:* try adding 1/2 teaspoon each of thyme, sage, and marjoram, plus a dash of salt.

ALL PHASES; SERVES APPROXIMATELY 8–10

Baked Turkey Roll-ups

Here's a fun dish that's quick and easy to fix and makes an interesting presentation. This recipe calls for whey protein powder for dredging.

4   5-ounce turkey breast cutlets
1/2 red pepper, julienned
1   carrot, julienned
1/2 small zucchini, julienned
1/2 small yellow squash, julienned
1   scoop (1 ounce) natural whey protein powder
1/2 teaspoon cumin
1/2 teaspoon garlic powder
1/2 teaspoon onion powder
1/4 teaspoon dried mustard
1   egg, beaten
     Juice of 1/2 lemon

Preheat oven to 400°F. Pound turkey cutlets between plastic wrap to 1/4-inch thickness. In a medium bowl, combine red pepper, carrot, zucchini, and yellow squash and mix well. Place a quarter of the veggie mixture at the end of each turkey cutlet and roll up. Secure with toothpicks. In a small bowl, combine whey powder, cumin, garlic powder, onion powder, and dried mustard. Dip rolled-up turkey cutlet in egg and then roll in whey powder mixture. Place turkey cutlets in non-stick baking pan and place in oven for 15 minutes or until meat juices run clear. Drizzle lemon juice over cutlets and serve.

Variation:
For phase 3: 1/2 teaspoon of salt may be added to the whey mixture.

ALL PHASES; SERVES 4

Dijon Turkey Cutlets

This dish is a delectable vehicle for the Ezekiel 4:9 bread crumbs. These bread crumbs provide a nutty, earthy flavor and are made from a sprouted grain recipe inspired by the Bible. Serve with Cinnamony Apple Sauce (page 248) and a baby green salad with one of the Fat Flush dressings.

4   5-ounce turkey cutlets
1/2 teaspoon prepared Dijon mustard
1   garlic clove, minced
1   cup Fat Flush Bread Crumbs (page 203)
1   teaspoon fresh parsley, chopped
1   egg, beaten

Pound the turkey cutlets to 1/4-inch thickness. Mix the bread crumbs, mustard, garlic, and parsley together in a mixing bowl. Dip the turkey cutlets in the egg. Then dip the cutlets into the bread crumbs. Cook the coated cutlets, a few at a time, in a nonstick skillet over medium heat until done (about 2–3 minutes per side). Remove and serve warm.

PHASES 2 AND 3; SERVES 4

Chicken à la Greco

Okay. For those of you who are following the Food Combination phase 3 recommendations in The Fat Flush Plan, *rest assured that yogurt does not seem to have the negative digestive impact of other dairy products like cheese and milk when used in a recipe with other animal-based proteins.*

	Zest of 1 lemon
	Juice of 1 lemon
3	tablespoons fresh parsley, chopped
1	teaspoon dried oregano
1/2	teaspoon dried marjoram
1/2	teaspoon dried thyme
2	garlic cloves, minced
1/2	teaspoon salt
2	tablespoons 1-2-3 Chicken Broth (page 222)
2	5-ounce chicken breasts, boned and skinned
1	tablespoon black olives, chopped
1/2	cup plain, whole milk yogurt

Mix together zest and 1/2 the juice of the lemon in a large bowl. Save the other half of the lemon juice. Add parsley, oregano, marjoram, thyme, garlic, salt, and broth. Add chicken, mix well, and let marinate for at least 2 hours in the refrigerator. Preheat broiler. Place chicken in a non-stick broiling pan and cook under broiler for 10 minutes. Turn and cook for another 10 minutes or until the juices from the chicken come out clear when pierced with a fork. While the chicken is cooking, blend the remaining juice of the lemon, olives, and yogurt in a small bowl. When chicken is done, serve with a spoonful of yogurt sauce.

PHASE 3; SERVES 2

Crispy Nonfried Chicken

You will be pleasantly surprised with the Fat Flush version of fried chicken. The herbs lend flavor and health value. Tarragon is a high source of potassium, while rosemary provides antioxidant power. Parsley is mineral-rich and garlic will fight off the vampires. Cinnamony Apple Sauce (page 248) goes well for dessert.

4   5-ounce chicken thighs, skinned
¾   cup 1-2-3 Chicken Broth (page 222)
1   tablespoon olive oil
1   cup toasted wheat germ or 1 cup Fat Flush Bread Crumbs (page 203)
1   teaspoon dried tarragon
1   teaspoon dried rosemary, crushed
1   teaspoon fresh parsley, chopped
1   teaspoon garlic powder
    Salt to taste

Preheat oven to 350°F. In a small bowl, place chicken broth and olive oil. In another bowl, mix together the wheat germ or bread crumbs, tarragon, rosemary, parsley, garlic powder, and salt. Dip the thighs, one at a time, in the broth-oil mixture. Then coat with the wheat germ or bread crumb–herb mixture. Bake in the oven until brown and cooked through, about 45–55 minutes.

PHASE 3; SERVES 4

Rosemary Cloves Grilled Chicken with Yogurt Sauce

Here's a special phase 3 dish that is very aromatic, thanks to the ground cloves.
(See the note about the yogurt in the Chicken à la Greco recipe on page 106.)

1   cup plain, whole milk yogurt
⅓   cup lemon juice
½   teaspoon ground cloves
2   garlic cloves, minced
4   5-ounce chicken breasts, boned and skinned
2   cups 1-2-3 Chicken Broth (page 222)
1   teaspoon dried rosemary, crushed
1   tablespoon fresh parsley, chopped

In a medium covered bowl, place yogurt, lemon juice, cloves, garlic, and chicken and let marinate refrigerated for at least 2 hours or overnight. Place broth and rosemary in a medium saucepan over high heat and boil until broth is reduced and thickened. Cool and set aside. Preheat broiler, or light a gas or charcoal grill. Remove chicken from marinade and broil for 8–10 minutes or place on grill for 10–15 minutes, turning occasionally. Reheat the reduced chicken broth in a small saucepan and add parsley. Transfer to a small bowl for serving. Remove chicken from broiler or grill and serve with the warm sauce.

PHASE 3; SERVES 4

BEEF, VEAL, AND LAMB

Burgers with Herbs

Sometimes you are in the mood for a good burger. These burgers are nicely spiced.

1½ pounds lean ground beef
1   tablespoon dried mustard
2   garlic cloves, minced
1   teaspoon cayenne
1   tablespoon fresh cilantro, chopped

Preheat broiler. Combine all ingredients and shape into patties. Broil on nonstick broiler pan until done.

Variations:
- *For phase 2:* add ½ teaspoon of mint to replace the cayenne.
- *For phase 3:* substitute dried horseradish for the mustard.

ALL PHASES; SERVES 4

Frankly Flank

The trick with this dish is to slice the meat thinly diagonally across the grain when you are getting ready to serve it, because flank steak can be a bit tough.

1–1½   pounds lean flank steak
1   teaspoon onion powder
1   teaspoon garlic powder
1   teaspoon dried mustard

Preheat broiler. Place flank steak in nonstick broiling pan. Sprinkle onion and garlic powders on top of steak. Broil for about 4–5 minutes on each side until done.

Variations:

- *For phase 3:* marinate in ½ cup sherry with 2 small minced garlic cloves and ¼ teaspoon ground ginger before broiling.
- *For phase 3 Special Occasions:* marinate in sherry, garlic, and ginger mixture with ½ teaspoon low-sodium wheat free tamari.

ALL PHASES; SERVES 4

Beef Stroganoff

A gourmet treat, this dish can be served with I Can't Believe It Isn't Garlicky Mashed Potatoes (page 142).

3   cups button mushrooms, sliced
1   cup shitake mushrooms, sliced
1   large onion, sliced
3   garlic cloves, minced
2   tablespoons plus 1 14-ounce can no-salt-added beef broth
1   pound flank steak, thinly sliced
2   tablespoons Fat Flush Catsup (page 206)
½   teaspoon garlic powder
     Tofu Sour Cream (see below)
1   medium spaghetti squash, as prepared in Fat Flush Spaghetti with
     Meat Sauce (page 114)

In a large skillet over medium heat, sauté button and shitake mushrooms, onion, and garlic cloves in 2 tablespoons of broth for 8 minutes or until onions are soft. Remove mushroom-onion mixture from skillet and set aside. Lightly brown flank steak in skillet for approximately 5 minutes. Add remaining broth, catsup, and garlic powder, cover, and simmer for 10 minutes. Return mushroom-onion mixture to skillet, add Tofu Sour Cream, mix well, bring to a boil, and cook for 1 minute. Serve over cooked spaghetti squash.

Tofu Sour Cream

1   12-ounce block silken, firm tofu
     Juice of 1 lemon
1   teaspoon apple cider vinegar
12   black olives

Place all ingredients in a blender and blend until smooth.

Variations:
* You may substitute mashed cauliflower for the spaghetti squash.
* *For phase 3:* add ½ teaspoon of salt after the garlic powder to the Beef Stroganoff.
* *For phase 3:* add a pinch of cardamom to the Tofu Sour Cream.

ALL PHASES; SERVES 4

Stuffed Cabbage

Here's a stuffed cabbage with a unique gingery flavor. Ginger is a warming herb, and its pungent, peppery taste stimulates digestion and increases circulation. Try this dish with Spicy Pumpkin (page 157).

8   large cabbage leaves, washed

¼   cup leek, finely chopped

1   teaspoon fresh ginger, grated, or pinch of dried ginger

½   pound ground lean beef

2   garlic cloves, minced

1   egg, lightly beaten

2   cups 1-2-3 Beef Broth (page 223)

8   toothpicks

2   tablespoons fresh parsley, chopped

In a large pot, cook cabbage in boiling water until soft enough to be used as wrapping. Gently remove cabbage from the hot water with a slotted spoon, refresh in cold water, and dry. In a medium skillet, sauté leek, ginger, beef, and garlic until the beef is cooked through. Add the egg to the meat and mix thoroughly for filling. Divide the filling into 8 portions, placing each portion in the middle of a cabbage leaf. Fold the two opposite sides of the leaf over the filling and roll up tightly, securing with toothpicks. Arrange the cabbage rolls in the skillet, add broth, and simmer for 20 minutes. Sprinkle with parsley.

ALL PHASES; SERVES 2

Fragrant Fat Flush Meatballs

The fennel—which is so good for your digestion—is the high note in these Fat Flush Meatballs. This dish is terrific over a medley of steamed veggies like zucchini, snow peas, summer squash, and string beans (see pages 127–129) or serve with Roasted Peppers with Garlic (page 140).

1   pound lean ground beef
1/2 cup cauliflower, diced
1½ cups purified water
1/3 cup onion, chopped
1   garlic clove, minced
1   15-ounce can no-salt-added Muir Glen Tomato Sauce
1/2 teaspoon ground fennel
1/4 teaspoon Stevia Plus

Preheat oven to 350°F. Mix beef, cauliflower, 1/2 cup water, onion, and garlic together. Shape into meatballs and place into baking dish. In a separate bowl, stir tomato sauce, 1 cup water, fennel, and Stevia Plus. Pour over the meatballs. Cover and bake for 45 minutes. Remove cover and bake for an additional 10–15 minutes or until done.

ALL PHASES; SERVES 4

Fat Flush Spaghetti with Meat Sauce

A wildly popular favorite, here's how to put spaghetti and meatballs together the Fat Flush way.

1	medium spaghetti squash
1	16-ounce can Muir Glen Tomato Puree
1	teaspoon ground fennel
1/4	teaspoon Stevia Plus
2	garlic cloves, crushed
1	pound lean ground beef
1/2	onion, chopped
1	cup mushrooms, sliced

Preheat oven to 350°F. Cut spaghetti squash in half lengthwise and scoop out the seeds. Place cut side down on a baking sheet and bake for 30 minutes. When spaghetti squash is cooked, use a fork to remove the flesh that forms spaghettilike strands. While the squash is cooking, mix beef, onion, and mushrooms together in a skillet. Cook over medium heat and until done. While the meat is cooking, put the tomato puree, fennel, Stevia Plus, and garlic in a 2-quart saucepan. Simmer over medium heat for 20 minutes. When the meat is cooked, add it to the sauce. Toss the spaghetti strands with the sauce and serve.

Variations:
- Substitute Fragrant Fat Flush Meatballs (page 113) for the meat sauce.
- *For phase 2:* add 1/2 teaspoon oregano and basil to the spices.

ALL PHASES; SERVES 4

Spiced Beef Over Spaghetti Squash

Another variation on the spaghetti and meatballs theme—you may try this if you have more time. It goes nicely with Glorious Greens (page 139) or Carrots and Snow Peas with Parsley (page 152) for phase 2.

2½ pounds beef rump (eye of round is best)

6   bay leaves

½   teaspoon ground cloves

2   medium onions, quartered

15   ounces no-salt-added tomato purée

1½ cups apple cider vinegar

1½ cups 1-2-3 Beef Broth (page 223)

3   stalks celery, cut into chunks

1   8-ounce can tomato paste

1   medium spaghetti squash, as prepared in Fat Flush Spaghetti with Meatballs (page 114)

Preheat oven to 400°F. Place the meat, bay leaves, cloves, onions, tomato purée, vinegar, broth, and celery in a roasting pan. Cook in oven for 20 minutes. Reduce temperature to 325°F, cover, and continue cooking for 3 hours. When meat is almost done, cook the spaghetti squash. When meat is tender, remove from roasting pan and cool. Remove bay leaves from the roasting pan. Place roasting pan on stove over medium heat and whisk in the tomato paste. Slice meat and serve over spaghetti squash, topped with sauce.

ALL PHASES; SERVES 8

Zucchini and Beef Delight

The zucchini is one vegetable with a lot of adaptability; it can be stuffed, sautéed, baked, and used in soups. In this recipe, the zucchini acts as a flavor carrier, absorbing the flavors and aromas of the cumin, cinnamon, cayenne, and turmeric. Serve over Kari's Marvelously Mashed Cauliflower (page 143) with Saucy Rhubarb (page 249) for dessert.

½   cup 1-2-3 Chicken Broth (page 222)
1   medium onion, diced
1   green pepper, sliced
4   garlic cloves, minced
4   small zucchini, cut into ¼-inch slices
1   pound lean ground beef
1   teaspoon ground cumin
½   teaspoon cinnamon
1   teaspoon cayenne
1   teaspoon ground turmeric
1   14½-ounce can no-salt-added diced tomatoes
2   tablespoons tomato paste
    Handful of fresh cilantro, chopped

In a large, nonstick skillet over medium heat, heat broth. Add onion, green pepper, garlic and zucchini and sauté until soft. Transfer vegetables onto plate and set aside. In the same nonstick skillet, brown beef, cumin, cinnamon, cayenne, and turmeric until beef is cooked through. Add cooked vegetables, diced tomatoes, and tomato paste to skillet. Heat through and add cilantro before serving.

Variation:
Ground turkey may be used instead of ground beef.

ALL PHASES; SERVES 4

Veal Medallions with Mushrooms and Garlic

This is good enough for company yet simple, fast, and healthy. The clean and fresh taste of Mashed Celery Root (page 144) is a good flavor balancer.

1   pound veal medallions, pounded to ⅛-inch thickness
½   cup 1-2-3 Beef Broth (page 223)
1   large onion, chopped
2   cups mushrooms, sliced
2   garlic cloves, minced

Brown veal with beef broth in a nonstick skillet. Remove veal from skillet and set aside. Sauté the onions, mushrooms, and garlic in remaining beef broth in the same skillet until tender. Return veal to skillet with onions, mushrooms, and garlic and heat through for about 1 minute or until done. Serve immediately.

ALL PHASES; SERVES 4

My Mother's Meatloaf

This dish is great for the family and for freezing. My mother Edith, who has been following the Fat Flushing principles for over ten years, tells me that the dried horseradish is the special ingredient in this recipe. Pungent and stimulating, horseradish is also a great source of both potassium and iron. It can increase circulation and perspiration, acting as a diuretic. Serve with I Can't Believe It Isn't Garlicky Mashed Potatoes (page 142).

1   tablespoon olive oil
2   pounds lean ground beef
1   cup Fat Flush bread crumbs (page 203)
¾   cup onions, chopped
1   teaspoon dried oregano
1   tablespoon dried horseradish
1   teaspoon dried mustard
½   cup Fat Flush Catsup (page 206)
2   eggs, beaten

Preheat oven to 350°F. Grease an 8- by 4-inch loaf pan with the olive oil. In a large bowl, mix the beef, bread crumbs, onions, oregano, horseradish, mustard, catsup, and eggs together. Shape into a loaf and place in the loaf pan. Bake for 1¼ hours or until done.

PHASE 3; SERVES 8

Coconutty Meatballs

The coconut milk is a saturated fat rich in antiviral substances that boost the immune system. Coconut milk and coconut oil are both making a comeback and certainly can be used in moderation in a balanced lifestyle program like phase 3 of Fat Flush.

1   pound lean ground beef
1   onion, finely chopped
2   garlic cloves, minced
1   egg, beaten
4   tablespoons plus ½ cup coconut milk, divided
1   teaspoon ground cumin
1   teaspoon ground coriander
¼   teaspoon cayenne
½   teaspoon salt
3   tablespoons fresh cilantro, chopped

Preheat broiler. In a large bowl, mix beef, onion, garlic, egg, 4 tablespoons of coconut milk, cumin, coriander, cayenne, and salt. Form into golf-ball–size meatballs and place on a nonstick broiling pan. Broil until meat is browned and no longer pink inside. Remove meatballs onto a serving dish and discard fat. Pour in remaining coconut milk making sure to dissolve all browned residues. Add cilantro, stirring until blended, and pour over meatballs. Serve immediately.

PHASE 3 SPECIAL OCCASION; SERVES 4

Sweet and Sour Beef

The date sugar provides the sweetness in this recipe—as well as fiber, potassium, and trace minerals.

2   pounds lean beef for stew, cubed
¼   cup 1-2-3 Beef Broth (page 223)
2   cups no-salt-added diced tomatoes
⅓   cup date sugar
⅓   cup apple cider vinegar
½   cup onion, chopped
3   whole cloves
1   bay leaf
1   green pepper, cut into thin strips

In a large skillet over medium heat, heat broth. Add beef and brown on all sides. Add tomatoes, date sugar, vinegar, onion, cloves, and bay leaf, blending well. Lower heat, cover, and simmer for 2 hours or until beef is tender. Add pepper strips and cook for 10 minutes. Remove cloves and bay leaf before serving.

PHASE 3 SPECIAL OCCASION; SERVES 4

Spiced Lamb à la Morocco

The delicate flavors of the allspice, ginger, and cinnamon will transport you to Morocco.

2   tablespoons plus 1½ cups 1-2-3 Chicken Broth (page 222), divided
1   onion, chopped
2   pounds boneless lamb, trimmed and cut into 1½-inch cubes
½   teaspoon ground anise
½   teaspoon ground ginger
1   16-ounce can no-salt-added peeled tomatoes
1   3-inch cinnamon stick
1   cup carrots, halved and cut into ½-inch pieces
2   cups yellow squash, cut into 1-inch cubes
1   cup celery, cut into ½-inch pieces
    Fresh parsley for garnish

Sauté onion in 2 tablespoons of broth in a skillet. Add lamb, anise, and ginger and cook until brown. Add tomatoes, additional broth, and cinnamon stick, cover, and cook over low heat for 40 minutes. Uncover, add carrots, squash, and celery and cook a further 15–20 minutes or until lamb and veggies are tender. Sprinkle with chopped parsley before serving.

PHASE 3; SERVES 8

Lamb Kebabs

A friend created this recipe and says that Asparagus with Lemon-Herb Dressing (page 145) is a tasty companion.

½   cup apple cider vinegar

¼   teaspoon cayenne

1½ teaspoon dried oregano, crushed

½   teaspoon dried rosemary, crushed

½   cup onion, minced

1   garlic clove, minced

1½ pounds lamb, trimmed and cut into 1½-inch cubes

8   whole mushrooms

1   medium red pepper, seeded and cut into 8 pieces

8   small, whole boiling onions, parboiled

4   skewers

In a medium bowl, combine the vinegar, cayenne, oregano, rosemary, onion, and garlic for a marinade and mix well. Add the lamb, making sure to coat evenly with marinade. Cover and let marinate in the refrigerator overnight. Remove lamb from marinade. Make kebabs by alternating the lamb with mushrooms, red peppers, and onions on the skewers. Cook over grill or barbecue for 15–20 minutes turning, the skewers repeatedly, until the meat is done and nicely browned.

PHASE 2 AND 3; SERVES 4

Lamb Chops Glazed with Apricot Preserves

This dish is so simple, it is sinful. You are sure to get many compliments on this.

8   baby lamb chops, trimmed of all visible fat
8   tablespoons unsweetened apricot preserves
½   teaspoon ground ginger

Preheat broiler. Place chops on nonstick broiling pan. In a small bowl, mix apricot preserves with ginger. Spread ½ of mixture over top of the chops. Broil for 5 minutes. Turn over and spread remaining preserves over other side. Broil another 5 minutes or until cooked through.

Variations:

- Substitute unsweetened peach preserves for the apricot preserves and replace ginger with (or add) a dash of cinnamon.
- In place of the apricot preserves and ginger, try marinating the lamb chops in ⅓ cup unsweetened pineapple juice with ½ tablespoon Fat Flush Curry Seasoning (page 204) and then broiling.

PHASE 3 SPECIAL OCCASION; SERVES 4

7 Vegetables

Rainbow-colored vegetables play a major role in Fat Flush—the more vibrant the pigment, the more packed with health-promoting antioxidants. The vegetable recipes contain lots of calcium-rich, dark, leafy greens (spinach and kale) that are also good sources of folic acid (which prevents birth defects) and vision protective lutein. Yellow-green selections include peas (phases 2 and 3) and corn (phase 3), which also contain lutein as well as zeaxanthin, another plant-based antioxidant which helps to prevent cataracts and macular degeneration—the most common cause of blindness in the elderly. You will find yellowish orange selections (like phase 2 acorn squash, sweet potatoes, and carrots) bursting with beta-carotene. And there are many dishes featuring tomatoes, cooked tomatoes, and tomato sauce—tasty sources of lycopene, the red compound that is a powerful aid in supporting prostate and breast health. The white-green vegetable choices such as onions, garlic, mushrooms, endive, leeks, and celery provide us with allicin and flavonoids which are cell protectors and strengthen immunity.

When it comes to veggies, think blue-purple (eggplant and cabbage), red, orange-yellow, and green. These veggies are best stored, by the way, loose or in plastic bags that are perforated so that the veggies can breathe. And store your veggies in a separate bin from fresh fruits. Many fruits like pears and apples, for instance, produce a ripening gas called ethylene which can alter the taste of vegetables

THE HEIRLOOM REVIVAL

When it comes to color, there is nothing more visually vibrant than heirloom vegetables. These veggies (and fruits, by the way) are making their way back onto America's tables. These are specialty vegetables with all their original genetic characteristics intact as were veggies before modern agriculture replaced them with hybrids that were designed to have a longer shelf life, were easier to ship, and were easier to process through machine harvesting.

The heirlooms are definitely more colorful and packed with higher nutritional values. Some kinds of heirloom corn, for example, are true powerhouses of protein—providing nearly three times the amount of protein of today's hybrid corn. Some kinds of heirloom apples are richer sources of vitamin C than your typical orange.

Today heirlooms can be found in upscale grocery stores, in farmers markets, and on roadside stands. Or you can grow your own from seeds, which are available in health food stores, at upscale grocery stores, or from seed supply companies on the Internet. The main reason for this renaissance, however, probably has nothing to do with nutrition or health. The taste of these heirlooms is simply out of this world.

Whether you are enjoying fresh, organic, or heirloom produce, the rule of thumb is simply this: If fresh or frozen are unavailable, than the next best are canned or jarred with no added salt. First and foremost, look for the words "no salt added" and/or "no sugar added" on the label for both canned and jarred veggies. When it comes to other additives or preservatives (such as EDTA, ascorbic acid, and citric acid, for example), the least amount the better, although these have no known toxicity.

By the way, Del Monte and Ready Pack Leafy Greens Blend have prewashed and precut fresh greens in plastic bags. So now there's really no excuse for *not* eating your greens because it doesn't get any easier than prewashed and ready cut! Spinach, chard, kale, collards, and turnip and mustard greens are a great source of folic acid and nondairy calcium on Fat Flush, as you may remember from *The Fat Flush Plan*.

From a practical standpoint, the best cooking news about vegetables is this: With a small, stainless steel steamer you can have maximum taste with a minimum of effort. The veggies can be crisply tender or firm and crunchy. When veggies are cooked this way, on the average, they take only 10–15 minutes. Of course, the tougher ones, like artichokes take longer.

So before you delve any further, take a look below at our Fat Flush Vegetable Steaming Guide. I know you will enjoy experimenting with the herbs and herb blends that can be used for each and every phase of the plan. Many of these herbs can single-handedly or in combination take an ordinary veggie from simple to sublime in minutes.

THE 3:1 HERB RATIO

Remember that when seasoning your veggies (or even main dishes for that matter) with herbs, the basic ratio for fresh to dried is 3:1. In other words, for dill you would replace 3 teaspoons or 1 tablespoon of fresh dill with 1 teaspoon of dried dill.

Any vegetable can be further accented with a drizzle of flaxseed oil, a baste of chicken, beef, or veggie broth, lemon juice, and herbs for phases 1 and 2. For phase 3, you can widen your taste horizons with a drizzle of olive, grape seed, or sesame oil for lifestyle eating and enjoyment. In phase 3, you can further experiment by also adding some crunch to your vibrant veggies in the form of toasted pine nuts, almonds, walnuts, filberts, and pumpkin and sunflower seeds to your vegetables—whether sautéed or steamed.

Insider Tip: When steaming veggies, use purified water. After the veggies are steamed, you can save this nutrient-rich water and add it to your ready-made or home-made broths for extra vitamins, minerals, and flavor.

Insider Tip: If steaming is not your thing, how about roasting your veggies in a hot oven. Roasting helps to potentize flavors in phase 2 and 3 favorites (think sweet potatoes) because the natural sugars caramelize.

THE FAT FLUSH VEGETABLE STEAMING GUIDE

VEGETABLE	STEAMING TIME
ARTICHOKES	
Globe, whole	45 minutes
INSIDER TIP:	Delicious with a sprinkling of lemon juice, basil, or thyme.
ASPARAGUS	
Whole	7–12 minutes
Tips	6–10 minutes
INSIDER TIP:	Bring out flavor with lemon zest, parsley, tarragon, or mustard.
BEANS	
Green, wax, or yellow	8–12 minutes
INSIDER TIP:	Flavor with a dash of coriander, basil, or garlic.
BEETS	
Whole	20–25 minutes
$\frac{1}{4}$-inch slices	3–5 minutes
INSIDER TIP:	A bit of cloves, ginger, or bay leaf really enhances flavor.
BROCCOLI	
Stalks, split	8–10 minutes
INSIDER TIP:	Try some mustard, garlic, or tarragon to heighten taste.
BRUSSELS SPROUTS	8–12 minutes
INSIDER TIP:	Delicious with garlic, basil, sage, or thyme.
CABBAGE	
Green, quartered	5–7 minutes
Green or red, shredded	3 minutes
INSIDER TIP:	Turmeric, mustard, or oregano will tickle your taste buds.

VEGETABLE	STEAMING TIME
CARROTS	
Whole	15–20 minutes
¼-inch slices	8–12 minutes
INSIDER TIP:	Please your palate with a sprinkling of dill, ginger, mint, or nutmeg.
CAULIFLOWER	
Whole	20–25 minutes
Florets	7–10 minutes
INSIDER TIP:	Try a sprinkling of cumin, rosemary, or marjoram.
CELERY	
Whole	8–12 minutes
Diced	3–7 minutes
INSIDER TIP:	Celery by itself acts as a spice to bring out the flavor of other veggies.
CORN	
On cob	5–8 minutes
Kernels	3–5 minutes
INSIDER TIP:	Add sweet basil. Sweet basil and cayenne powder can perk things up.
EGGPLANT	
Sliced	8–10 minutes
INSIDER TIP:	Delicious with garlic, oregano, basil, or marjoram.
KALE	3–7 minutes
INSIDER TIP:	Garlic and lemon are perky taste enhancers.
KOHLRABI	
Whole	10–15 minutes
Sliced	3–7 minutes
INSIDER TIP:	Similar to kale, kohlrabi goes well with garlic and lemon.

VEGETABLE	STEAMING TIME
OKRA	
Whole	10–12 minutes
Sliced	3–6 minutes
INSIDER TIP:	Try a sprinkling of dill or basil to heighten taste.
ONIONS	5–8 minutes
INSIDER TIP:	Delicious with a sprinkling of cumin, oregano, thyme, or nutmeg.
SNOW PEAS	3–5 minutes
INSIDER TIP:	There is nothing like minced garlic or crushed mint to bring out the flavor.
SPINACH	3–5 minutes
INSIDER TIP:	Try with garlic, basil, nutmeg, or marjoram for a taste treat.
SQUASH, YELLOW	
Whole	15–25 minutes
¼-inch slices	8–10 minutes
INSIDER TIP:	Great with a sprinkling of cloves, fennel, ginger, or nutmeg.
SWISS CHARD	3–5 minutes
INSIDER TIP:	Try with a garlic clove, lemon zest, or fennel.
TOMATOES	
Whole	5–8 minutes
½-inch slices	3–5 minutes
INSIDER TIP:	Fennel, anise, basil, or oregano are a tomato's best friend.
ZUCCHINI	
Whole	8–12 minutes
¼-inch slices	3–6 minutes
INSIDER TIP:	Garlic or basil bring out the flavor.

Spinach Toss

A lovely side salad for any Fat Flush entrée of your choice, spinach is not only a terrific source of eye-nourishing lutein but is rich in potassium as well.

4   cups fresh spinach, shredded
1   cup jícama, cut into thin strips
½   cup mushrooms, sliced
2   tablespoons flaxseed oil
1   tablespoon lemon juice
¼   teaspoon Stevia Plus (optional)
⅛   teaspoon garlic powder

In a large salad bowl, combine spinach, jícama, and mushrooms and toss lightly. Mix flaxseed oil, lemon juice, Stevia Plus, and garlic powder in a jar, cover, and shake well. Pour dressing over the salad and toss lightly.

ALL PHASES; SERVES 4

Broccoli-Cauliflower Salad

Both cauliflower and broccoli belong to the cruciferous vegetable family and are rich in sulfurlike compounds that support the detoxification process. I love this salad with Limey Chicken (page 95).

4   cups cauliflower florets
4   cups broccoli florets
2   tablespoons apple cider vinegar
4   tablespoons flaxseed oil
1   garlic clove, minced
2   tablespoons scallions, finely chopped
½   teaspoon dried mustard

In a steamer, place the cauliflower and broccoli and steam until just under-cooked, about 6 minutes. Transfer to a bowl and let cool. In a small bowl, blend vinegar, oil, garlic, scallions, and mustard. Pour the dressing over the cauliflower and broccoli and toss.

Variation:
For phase 3: serve with 4 tablespoons of slivered almonds.

ALL PHASES; SERVES 4

Jícama Slaw

Jícama is definitely a Fat Flush favorite! It is a crunchy alternative to cabbage and tastes similar to water chestnuts—only sweeter. Jícama is quite delicious when served raw. This slaw is perfect for packing with lunches. It's a terrific side with any fish dish but my choice would be Crispy Nonfried Fish (page 94).

12 ounces jícama, peeled and cut into thin strips
1   red onion, thinly sliced
1   carrot, grated
1   cucumber, cut into thin strips
1   cup parsley, chopped
1/2 cup apple cider vinegar
1/2 teaspoon dill
3   tablespoons flaxseed oil
3   garlic cloves, minced
    Juice of 1 lemon

In a large bowl, place jícama, onion, carrot, and cucumber and set aside. In a jar, put parsley, vinegar, dill, flaxseed oil, garlic, and lemon juice and shake well. Pour the dressing over the jicama mix and toss lightly.

Variations:
- Add 1/2 sliced whole fennel bulb for an intriguing taste sensation and substitute lime juice for the lemon.
- *For phase 3:* try adding toasted pumpkin seeds or sunflower seeds to the slaw.

ALL PHASES; SERVES 4

Eggplant Salad

Eggplant is part of the Solanaceae family of veggies, which may have potential as major disease fighters. A decent source of potassium, I like this dish with a simple turkey burger or any kind of beef or fish or with lamb kabobs.

2   eggplants
1   garlic clove
4   tablespoons flaxseed oil
1   tomato, diced
2   tablespoons onion, minced
2   tablespoons parsley, chopped
1   tablespoon apple cider vinegar

Preheat oven to 350°F. Place eggplants on a nonstick baking dish and bake for about 1 hour. Cool, peel, and dice eggplants and set aside. In the meantime, rub a salad bowl with the garlic clove and then discard the garlic. Place diced eggplant in salad bowl and add oil, tomato, onion, and parsley. Sprinkle the vinegar over the mixture and toss well. Chill before serving.

ALL PHASES; SERVES 4

Simply Grilled Mushrooms and Onions

This is a wonderful side dish to accent the beef entrées or even a hearty burger. In fact, I like this dish as a topping for my scrambled eggs.

¼ cup 1-2-3 Chicken or Beef Broths (page 222 or page 223)
8 ounces mushrooms, sliced
3 onions, sliced
1 garlic clove, minced
1 teaspoon lemon juice

In a medium skillet, heat broth over medium-high heat. Add mushrooms, onions, and garlic. Cook until onions are translucent and tender. Add lemon juice. Serve.

ALL PHASES; SERVES 2

Fat Flush Ratatouille

This simple veggie dish complements and dresses up plain broiled fish, chicken, or beef. I serve it most often as a side with Chicken with Dill (page 98) and even eat the leftovers with Crispy Potato Skins (page 166).

½   cup 1-2-3 Vegetable Broth (page 221)
¼   cup scallions, chopped
2   garlic cloves, minced and divided
1   pound zucchini cut into ½-inch slices
8   ounces Muir Glen Peeled Tomatoes
¼   teaspoon cayenne
1   tablespoon fresh parsley, chopped

In a large, covered saucepan, sauté scallions and 1 garlic clove in broth until lightly browned. Add zucchini and cook until tender. Add tomatoes, cayenne, and parsley, cooking over low heat and stirring occasionally for about 30–40 minutes. Add remaining garlic clove and cook uncovered for about 7 minutes.

Variation:

For phases 2 and 3: add ½ teaspoon dried basil and ½ teaspoon dried oregano with the cayenne.

ALL PHASES; SERVES 4

Carrot Burdock Stir Sauté

This is a very therapeutic as well as tasty dish. In Asian medicine the burdock is a revered blood cleanser and blood builder. It is found in many mainstream grocery stores, health food stores, or Asian markets. This dish is also good for your reproductive system.

4   tablespoons 1-2-3 Vegetable Broth (page 221)
2   medium burdocks, cut into thinly sliced shavings
4   small carrots, cut into thinly sliced shavings
    Dash of dried ginger
    Fresh parsley for garnish

In a large skillet, heat the broth over medium-high heat. Sauté burdock, carrots, and ginger for about 4 minutes or until tender-crisp. Serve warm and garnish with fresh parsley.

Variation:
For Special Occasion: add 1/4 teaspoon tamari.

ALL PHASES; SERVES 4

Dilly Okra

I am a big fan of okra. Lightly steamed (see Steaming Chart on page 129), it can be eaten just like green beans and makes a wonderful natural thickener for stews and soups. Plus, it has the added health benefits of easing constipation and lubricating the intestinal tract. Serve with Simply Baked Fish (page 85).

1½ cups okra, cut into ½-inch lengths and steamed
½   cup tomatoes, chopped
1   teaspoon dried dill

Put the okra, tomatoes, and dill in a pot and simmer for 5 minutes.

ALL PHASES; SERVES 4

Glorious Greens

Many people don't realize how calcium-rich green, leafy veggies really are! Choose from kale, collards, spinach, chard, and escarole. These glorious greens will do any entrée proud.

2   pounds assorted greens, trimmed and cleaned
2   cups purified water
¼   cup 1-2-3 Chicken Broth (page 222)
1   onion, sliced
2   garlic cloves, minced
    Juice of 1 lemon
4   tablespoons flaxseed oil

Place greens in a pot and add water to cover. Bring to a quick boil and then lower heat, simmer, cooking greens until barely tender, about 5–8 minutes depending upon toughness of greens. Drain, chop, and set aside. Heat broth in saucepan and sauté onion and garlic over low heat until tender. Quickly add greens to saucepan, reducing heat to low, and cook greens until tender. Dish greens into a bowl; add lemon juice and flaxseed oil and toss. Serve warm or at room temperature.

ALL PHASES; SERVES 4

Roasted Peppers with Garlic

Like the Simply Grilled Mushrooms and Onions (page 135), I personally enjoy this dish with eggs. I know you will enjoy it with Fragrant Fat Flush Meatballs (page 113).

4   large bell peppers (combination of colors), halved, seeded, and
    membranes removed
8   garlic cloves
2   cups purified boiled water
1   tablespoon flaxseed oil
½   cup parsley, chopped
½   cup scallions, chopped

Preheat broiler. Broil peppers on nonstick baking sheet, turning constantly
    until skin has browned. Remove the peppers and set aside in a paper
    bag for about 15 minutes. Peel skin from peppers and cut into long
    thin strips. Dry thoroughly with paper towels. Place garlic in a bowl
    with boiled water for 15 minutes. Cool and remove skins. Place garlic,
    oil, parsley, and scallions in a blender and blend to make a paste. Toss
    paste with peppers and refrigerate for 1 hour before serving.

ALL PHASES; SERVES 4

Brussels Sprouts with Curry

Brussels sprouts really did originate in Brussels, Belgium. They contribute many disease-fighting chemicals to the diet and are a fair source of beta-carotene, which is so helpful for immunity. They go well with just about any fish, meat, or poultry entrée.

1   pound Brussels sprouts, trimmed of outside leaves
1   cup 1-2-3 Chicken Broth (page 222)
1   medium onion, finely chopped
2   teaspoons Fat Flush Curry Seasoning (page 204)

Put all ingredients into a medium-sized pot. Bring to a quick boil, then simmer for about 15 minutes or until liquid cooks down. As liquid starts to thicken, gently coat Brussels sprouts with liquid glaze on all sides. Serve warm.

Variation:

Instead of the Brussels sprouts, try other members of the cancer-fighting cruciferous food family like broccoli, cauliflower, and cabbage.

ALL PHASES; SERVES 4

I Can't Believe It Isn't Garlicky Mashed Potatoes

The cauliflower is the special ingredient here, and you won't even miss potatoes if you are on phases 1 and 2. Mashing these "potatoes" with the peppers in a food processor (or blender) yields a pretty "confetti" effect—a perfect company dish! Serve with Beef Stroganoff (page 111) or My Mother's Meatloaf (page 118).

1   small onion, chopped
1/2 red pepper, chopped
1/2 yellow pepper, chopped
1/4 cup 1-2-3 Chicken Broth (page 222)
2   cups cooked cauliflower, diced
1/4 teaspoon dried dill
1/2 teaspoon garlic, minced

In a nonstick skillet, sauté onion and green pepper in broth for about 5 minutes over medium heat. Add cauliflower and toss until heated through. Add dill and garlic. Transfer to a food processor (or blender) and puree, adding an additional tablespoon of chicken broth to achieve a smooth consistency. Serve hot.

ALL PHASES; SERVES 2–3

Kari's Marvelously Mashed Cauliflower

This recipe has become the Fat Flush answer to mashed potatoes and white rice. It appears as an accompaniment to several of the entrees like Fat Flush Shepherd's Pie (page 79).

1   medium head cauliflower, cut into florets
1   cup purified water
2   garlic cloves, minced
1   teaspoon fresh chives, chopped
½   teaspoon onion powder
½   teaspoon fresh parsley, chopped
1   tablespoon 1-2-3 Chicken or Beef Broth (page 222 or page 223)

In a medium pot, place cauliflower with water and bring to a quick boil. Lower heat to simmer and cover. Cook for an additional 12 minutes or until soft. Drain, transfer cauliflower to a bowl, and mash. Blend in garlic, chives, onion powder, parsley, and broth with the mashed cauliflower. Serve hot.

ALL PHASES; SERVES 2

Mashed Celery Root

Celery root, or celeriac, looks like an aged, brown turnip. It is a natural diuretic and digestive aid and supports the lymph and nervous systems. Serve with Veal Medallions with Mushrooms and Garlic (page 117).

4   medium celery root (celeriac), skin removed and cut into ½-inch
    cubes
4   garlic cloves, minced
½   teaspoon onion powder
½   cup 1-2-3 Chicken or Beef Broth (page 222 or page 223)
1   tablespoon fresh parsley, chopped

Place all ingredients in a nonstick saucepan and bring to a quick boil.
Reduce heat, cover, and simmer for 25 minutes, stirring occasionally.
Add more broth if needed. Remove from heat and mash. Sprinkle
with parsley for garnish.

ALL PHASES; SERVES 2

Asparagus with Flaxy Lemon-Herb Dressing

A potent natural diuretic, asparagus is a source of carotenoids and vitamin E. Serve with broiled lamb chops or Lamb Kebobs (page 122).

1   pound asparagus spears, trimmed
    Juice and zest of 1 lemon
¼   cup flaxseed oil
¼   cup apple cider vinegar
1   garlic clove, minced
1   tablespoon each—chopped chives, chopped fresh dill, and
    chopped fresh parsley

Blanch asparagus spears in large pot of boiling water for 5 minutes or until tender but not mushy. Plunge spears in ice water to cool quickly. Then drain. Add remaining ingredients in a small bowl and whisk together for dressing. Drizzle lemon-flaxseed dressing over asparagus before serving.

Variation:

For true parsley lovers, you may use 2 tablespoons of parsley to replace the chives and dill.

ALL PHASES; SERVES 4

Green Beans with Garlic and Spice

Green beans are delightfully flavorful when enhanced with garlic, turmeric, cumin, cayenne, and jalapeños (for those who like to turn up the heat). Serve as a side dish with lamb or beef.

1 cup 1-2-3 Chicken Broth (page 222), divided
3 garlic cloves, thinly sliced
2 small jalapeño peppers, seeds removed, minced (optional)
1 teaspoon turmeric
2 teaspoons cumin
1/8 teaspoon cayenne
1 pound whole green beans, trimmed
  Lemon juice for drizzling

Heat 1/2 cup broth in nonstick pan. Add garlic, jalapeños, turmeric, cumin, and cayenne and cook until the garlic turns golden, about 3 minutes. Add the green beans and remaining 1/2 cup broth and stir well. Cover and cook over medium heat, stirring occasionally for 5–6 minutes or until beans are tender. Drizzle with lemon juice and serve.

Variation:
You can add 1 package of frozen pearl onions, thawed, to add a sophisticated flair.

ALL PHASES; SERVES 4

Green Beans Oregano

The health-enhancing oregano in this dish will increase antioxidant levels 3 to 20 times more than other herbs. And Green Beans Oregano is simple and tasty, too.

1   pound green beans, sliced
½   cup purified water
½   teaspoon dried oregano

In a heavy saucepan, place green beans with water. Add oregano and cook uncovered until beans are crisp-tender, about 12 minutes. Drain well and serve.

ALL PHASES; SERVES 4

Caramelized Onions

A perfect partner with the Eggplant Bake (page 70), the sweetness of the onions also complements lean steak and hamburgers.

½ to 1   cup 1-2-3 Vegetable Broth (page 221)
4   large yellow onions, thinly sliced
4   tablespoons apple cider vinegar
¼   teaspoon Stevia Plus
1   tablespoon fresh cilantro, chopped

Heat 1/2 cup broth in nonstick pan. Add the onions and cook over medium heat for 30 minutes or until very tender. Add more broth as needed to keep from sticking. Stir in vinegar and Stevia Plus and cook for 10 more minutes or until onions are browned. Add cilantro before serving.

Variation:
After cooking, try drizzling with flaxseed oil for a buttery taste.

ALL PHASES; SERVES 4

Tangy Pickled Cauliflower

To keep the Indian theme and aromatic spices flowing, try this veggie side dish with Chicken Stir-Fry with a Touch of Turmeric (page 75). This recipe is courtesy of Kari Wheaton—the mashed cauliflower creator.

1   tablespoon 1-2-3 Chicken Broth (p. 222)
3   teaspoons Fat Flush Curry Seasoning (page 204)
1   teaspoon fresh ginger, minced
1   garlic clove, minced
1   stalk celery, minced
1   head cauliflower, broken into florets
1   cup purified water
1½ cups apple cider vinegar
1   teaspoon Stevia Plus
½   teaspoon dried dill

Cook the curry seasoning, ginger, garlic, and celery in broth in a nonstick pan over medium heat for 2 minutes. Add the cauliflower florets to the pan and toss to coat. Cook the cauliflower for 5 minutes or until slightly tender. In a large glass container, combine the water, vinegar, Stevia Plus, and dill. Place the spiced cauliflower into the container with the other ingredients. Store in the refrigerator for 1 week to allow flavors to develop before eating.

ALL PHASES; SERVES 4

Leeks with Garlic and Mustard

This simple dish cannot go wrong when paired with poultry, beef, or veal.

1   cup 1-2-3 Chicken Broth (page 222)
4   leeks, washed and cut in half lengthwise, then into ¼-inch strips at
    a diagonal
1   garlic clove, chopped
1   tablespoon fresh parsley, chopped
2   tablespoons apple cider vinegar
½   teaspoon dried mustard

Bring broth to a boil in a nonstick skillet on medium-high heat. Add leeks
    and garlic to the broth, cover, and simmer until leeks are tender, about
    10–12 minutes. Remove from heat, drain, transfer to large bowl, and
    stir in parsley, vinegar, and dried mustard. Ready to serve.

Variation:

Try this dish tossed with chopped hard-boiled eggs for a quick starter to a
lunch or dinner.

ALL PHASES; SERVES 4

Gingered Asparagus

This warming veggie dish goes well with salmon—especially Salmon Cakes (page 87).

1   pound asparagus spears, washed and dried
2   teaspoons fresh ginger, grated
2   garlic cloves, minced
2   teaspoons fresh parsley, chopped
¼   cup 1-2-3 Chicken Broth (page 222)
2   teaspoons fresh lemon juice
1   tablespoon flaxseed oil (optional)

In a medium-sized bowl, toss the asparagus with ginger, garlic, and parsley and let stand for 20 minutes or longer. Bring broth to a quick boil in a nonstick skillet. Add asparagus and herbs to the broth, lower heat, and sauté for 12 minutes, turning the asparagus occasionally until the spears are just tender. Remove onto a serving dish and drizzle with lemon juice and flaxseed oil.

Variation:
For phases 2 and 3: add 1 teaspoon dried mint to the seasonings.

ALL PHASES; SERVES 4

Carrots and Snow Peas with Parsley

Carrots and snow peas team up with basil to provide an interesting flavor twist with Spiced Beef over Spaghetti Squash (page 115).

2   garlic cloves, minced
4   carrots, cut into thin strips
2   tablespoons 1-2-3 Chicken Broth (page 222)
¼   pound snow peas, strings removed from both sides
1   tablespoon fresh parsley, chopped

Sauté garlic and carrots in broth in a nonstick skillet for 7–10 minutes. Add snow peas and cook for about 2 minutes or until crisp-tender. Remove from heat. Stir in parsley and serve.

Variation:

For phases 2 and 3: 1 tablespoon of fresh basil may replace the fresh parsley.

ALL PHASES; SERVES 4

Puréed Sweet Potatoes

Vegetable purées are a great way to add color-packed antioxidants to the plate. They are easy to make, and your guests will be impressed. This basic purée recipe can be used for any vegetable, but the ones that work the best are Brussels sprouts, asparagus, eggplant, and red pepper for phase 1, rutabagas, yams, and butternut squash for phase 2, and chestnuts for phase 3. I like this dish with Roast Turkey with Lemon, Garlic, and Fennel (page 103).

2   small sweet potatoes, skinned, baked, and mashed
½   cup 1-2-3 Chicken Broth (page 222)
⅛   teaspoon ground cumin
     Fresh parsley sprigs for garnish

Purée the sweet potatoes, broth, and cumin in a blender. Garnish with parsley sprigs.

Variation:
For phase 3: a dash of nutmeg would be divine.

PHASES 2 AND 3; SERVES 2

Red Cabbage with Chestnuts

This cabbage dish can be served hot or cold with the Artichoke Frittata (page 69).

¼ cup 1-2-3 Chicken Broth (p. 222)
2   tablespoons onion, diced
4   cups red cabbage, shredded
¼ cup apple cider vinegar
     Pinch of turmeric
12   chestnuts, roasted and peeled, or reconstituted from dried

Sauté onions in broth over medium heat in a nonstick skillet. Add cabbage, vinegar, and turmeric, and mix gently. Cover, lower heat, and simmer until cabbage is tender, about 20 minutes, stirring occasionally. Blend in chestnuts, cook through another 5 minutes. Serve hot or cold.

PHASE 3; SERVES 4

Zucchini Cheese Bake

This dish can be combined with a couple of eggs for breakfast.

2   cups zucchini, thinly sliced
4   ounces Swiss cheese, cubed
2   tablespoons Parmesan cheese, grated
2   tablespoon fresh parsley, chopped
1   tablespoon chives, chopped
½   cup Fat Flush Bread Crumbs (page 203)

Preheat oven to 350°F. In a nonstick baking dish, in layers, spread ⅓ of the zucchini, Swiss and Parmesan cheese, parsley, and chives. Repeat process twice and top with bread crumbs. Bake uncovered for 30 minutes; the bread crumbs should be golden brown, and not burnt.

Variation:

No zucchini? Summer squash, broccoli, and asparagus will work quite well, too.

PHASE 3; SERVES 4

Cauliflower and Peas in Yogurt

This Indian-style veggie dish is perfect for lacto-ovo vegetarians and combines well with any tempeh or tofu dish.

1   cauliflower, cut into florets
1   cup peas, thawed
¼   teaspoon ground cumin
¼   teaspoon ground coriander
    Dash of ground nutmeg
1   tablespoon lemon juice
3   tablespoons cilantro, chopped
1   cup plain whole milk yogurt
    Salt to taste (optional)

Steam cauliflower for 10 minutes, until tender. Place in a serving bowl. Steam peas for 5 minutes until cooked. Add to cauliflower, with the remaining ingredients. Mix well and chill before serving.

PHASE 3; SERVES 4

Spicy Pumpkin

An excellent source of the antioxidant beta-carotene, pumpkins are very versatile—their seeds and pulp are Fat Flush–friendly. The fiery cayenne in this recipe is complimented by the gingery flavor of Stuffed Cabbage (page 112).

1   pound pumpkin, peeled, deseeded, and cut into ½-inch-wide lengths
2   tablespoons olive oil
½   teaspoon cayenne
½   teaspoon lemon zest
2   tablespoon fresh lemon juice
1   tablespoon fresh basil, chopped

Cook pumpkin in boiling water for 3–5 minutes (or alternatively steam pumpkin for 5 minutes) until just soft. Drain and put the pumpkin on a serving plate. In a small bowl, mix together the oil, cayenne, lemon zest, and lemon juice. Pour mixture over the pumpkin. Garnish with basil before serving.

PHASE 3; SERVES 4

Sweet Potato Delight

This is easy and deceptively rich. It goes great with turkey.

4   small sweet potatoes, baked
1/3   cup unsweetened pineapple juice
1   egg, beaten
1/4   teaspoon ground cloves
1/4   teaspoon ground cinnamon
1/4   teaspoon ground nutmeg

Preheat oven to 350°F. Peel sweet potatoes (or leave skin on if you prefer). Mash and blend in pineapple juice. Add in egg and spices and beat until foamy. Pour into a casserole dish sprayed with nonstick cooking spray. Bake for about 35 minutes.

Variations:
- Top with shredded coconut.
- Top with toasted, ground flaxseeds.

PHASE 3 SPECIAL OCCASION; SERVES 4

8 Snacks

Snacks are not just an afterthought. On Fat Flush they are as important as regular meals because they keep blood sugar levels steady. In fact, as many of you already know from *The Fat Flush Plan,* you must eat about every 3 hours to keep blood sugar levels steady, which avoids the over-production of the fat-promoting hormone insulin at the next meal. This section provides a nice selection of pâtés and spreads which make perfect snacks that can be prepared ahead of time and kept in the fridge. Many of these, by the way, can be used as appetizers or hors d'oeuvres.

In addition to the fresh Fat Flush fruits for each phase and the snack recipes that follow, consider trying these easy snack ideas to satisfy the between meal munchies:

SPEEDY SNACKS FOR ALL PHASES

- Precut veggies such as zucchini, broccoli and cauliflower florets, string beans, radishes, baby asparagus spears, and carrots in apple cider vinegar/flaxseed oil marinade
- 1 steamed artichoke dipped in Homemade Salsa (page 207)
- Jícama rounds sprinkled with fresh lime juice and a dash of cayenne
- Celery sticks and red pepper slices
- Chicken broth with chopped spinach or escarole sprinkled with ground or milled flaxseeds
- Red and yellow cherry and pear tomatoes with a squeeze of lemon
- Button mushrooms with a dash of garlic powder and onion powder
- Artichoke hearts with black olives
- Sliced cucumbers with apple cider vinegar and dill
- Fennel stalks with lemon juice
- Beef broth soup with sliced mushrooms and onions
- Sliced apple or nectarine rolled in toasted ground or milled flaxseeds with cinnamon
- Red, yellow, green, and orange bell peppers cut into strips
- Snow peas split open and spread with tofu and toasted ground or milled flaxseeds

- Water chestnuts sprinkled with fresh lemon juice and a dash of ground ginger
- Cascadian Farms Reduced Sodium Kosher Dill Pickles (rinsed well under running water)
- Stuffed celery ribs with mashed tofu, garlic powder, onion powder, and a dash of cayenne

PHASES 2 AND 3

- 1 Fat Flush Tortilla with chopped eggs, onions, and flaxseed oil
- 1 slice Fat Flush French Toast (page 62)
- 1 slice Health Seed Spelt toast drizzled with flaxseed oil
- 1 small yam sprinkled with toasted ground or milled flaxseeds
- 1/2 cup baked butternut or acorn squash slices with cinnamon
- Sliced tomato with flaxseed oil, oregano, and basil

PHASE 3

- 2 tablespoons toasted pumpkin seeds with a dash of cumin, coriander, and turmeric
- 1 tablespoon almond butter with cantaloupe chunks
- 1 tablespoon peanut butter on apple slices
- 1/2 mashed avocado with lemon juice, 1/2 teaspoon dried dill, and handful of blue corn chips
- 1 cup plain yogurt with 1/2 cup mixed melon chunks and chopped walnuts
- 1 cup plain yogurt with pomegranate seeds and slivered almonds
- 1 slice Swiss cheese with sliced tomatoes
- Endive leaves with 1 ounce sliced cheddar cheese
- 3 cups air-popped popcorn with flaxseed oil
- 1 small ear of corn on the cob with flaxseed oil
- 1 baked corn tortilla with Homemade Salsa (page 207)
- 1/2 banana rolled in toasted ground or milled flaxseeds with cardamom
- Frozen grapes (to freeze grapes, simply pop fresh grapes into an airtight container and freeze until solid)
- Frozen banana with dash of cinnamon (to freeze banana, peel a ripe banana and pop in an airtight container, freezing until solid)
- Snow peas split open and spread with 1/2 cup cottage cheese and a dash of Fat Flush Curry Seasoning (page 204)
- 1/2 cup ricotta cheese blended with 1/2 teaspoon lemon zest and 1 teaspoon Flora-Key
- Blanched baby squashes hollowed out and stuffed with fresh dill and cream cheese mixture

SPECIAL OCCASION

- 1 cup yogurt with 1/2 to 1 teaspoon blackstrap molasses, 1/4 teaspoon vanilla extract, and 1 tablespoon toasted ground or milled flaxseeds
- 1 cup hot coconut milk soup with sliced mushrooms, scallions, and lime
- 1 cup plain yogurt with 1 teaspoon honey, 3 tablespoons wheat germ, and 1/2 banana
- 1 fig stuffed with goat cheese and broiled
- Kiwi slices rolled in toasted ground flaxseeds and sprinkled with unsweetened shredded coconut
- 1 cup berries with whipped cream sweetened with Stevia Plus
- 1/2 grapefruit dabbed with 1 teaspoon honey and broiled for 3 minutes

RECIPES

Fat Flush Pickles

One of my premiere Fat Flush secrets is this: When you crave something sweet, satisfy that craving with something sour. And what could be better than these easy homemade pickles. These are great snacks—you can actually eat all of them in one sitting if you like, and they can be used sliced in salads and to accompany burgers.

8   cucumbers, cut into spears
1   cup apple cider vinegar
1   garlic clove, minced
2   teaspoons fresh dill
    Dash of turmeric

In a medium bowl, blend cucumbers, vinegar, garlic, dill, and turmeric. Cover, refrigerate for at least 6 hours and enjoy.

ALL PHASES; SERVES 4

Spinach Stuffed Mushrooms

This is a great party food, not to mention a quick and easy snack for you to pack and take with you.

1 10-ounce package frozen spinach, thawed and drained
1 egg yolk
1 garlic clove, minced
12 large white mushrooms, cleaned and stemmed

Heat oven to 350°F. Spray a small baking sheet with nonstick cooking spray. In a large bowl, mix spinach, egg yolk, and garlic. Stuff each mushroom with spinach mixture and place on baking sheet. Bake for 15–25 minutes or until mixture is firm to the touch. Serve hot.

Variations:

- *For phase 2:* add 1/2 teaspoon basil and oregano to stuffing mix.
- *For phase 3:* add 1/2 teaspoon nutmeg and 1/4 cup chopped walnuts to stuffing mix.

ALL PHASES; SERVES 4

Marinated Mushrooms

Well worth the effort, these marinated mushrooms are very satisfying. The apple cider vinegar marinade is milder and mellower than marinades made with other types of vinegars. It adds a fresh tang to the mushrooms. This snack is surprisingly filling.

½	teaspoon ground cumin
¼	teaspoon crushed fennel
½	teaspoon ground coriander
½	teaspoon onion powder
½	teaspoon garlic powder
1	garlic clove, thinly sliced
1	stalk celery, minced
1	bay leaf
½	teaspoon dried dill
¼	cup purified water
¼	cup apple cider vinegar
1	pound small, whole button mushrooms or large mushrooms, quartered
	Juice of 1 lemon
¼	cup flaxseed oil

In a saucepan, combine everything but the mushrooms, lemon juice, and flaxseed oil, and bring to a boil. Reduce heat, cover, and simmer for about 5 minutes. Add mushrooms, return to boil, reduce heat, then simmer another 5 minutes. Remove from stove and remove bay leaf. Let cool and add lemon juice and flaxseed oil. Place all ingredients in a glass jar, refrigerate, and let marinate for at least 1 hour. Serve cold.

ALL PHASES; SERVES 4

Peppy Mushrooms

This is a quick-fix nibble that will keep in the fridge for days.

¼ cup apple cider vinegar
2   tablespoons flaxseed oil
½ teaspoon cayenne
¼ teaspoon ground cloves
¼ teaspoon ground cumin
    Dash of coriander
1   pound small button mushrooms, stems removed

In a small bowl, combine everything but the mushrooms. Pour over mushrooms, cover, and refrigerate overnight. When ready to serve, drain and serve mushrooms with toothpicks.

ALL PHASES; SERVES 4

Crispy Potato Skins

I bet you thought potato skins were forever off limits on Fat Flush. The most nutritious part of the potato is right beneath the skin. High levels of vital trace minerals such as selenium, chromium, manganese, and potassium can be found there, not to mention vitamin C. Just make sure to remove any sprouts or green-ish color from the skins before you bake. I find that organic potatoes are less likely to contain these undesirable elements. Crispy Potato Skins can be topped with Homemade Salsa (page 207) or Cran-Jewel Catsup (page 209).

4   large potatoes, well scrubbed, for baking

Preheat oven to 400°F. Pierce potatoes with a fork and bake for about 1 hour or until potatoes are done inside. Remove and let cool. Scoop out the white inside part of the potato and transfer the skins to a nonstick baking sheet sprayed with nonstick cooking spray. Place the skins back in the oven for another 12 minutes or until they are crispy.

Variations:
- Top with Minty Dill Pesto (page 213) or Basil Pesto (page 214).
- You can sprinkle the skins with a tablespoon of Parmesan or melt a slice of Swiss or cheddar cheese.

PHASE 3; SERVES 4

Crab and Lime Quiche

This is also good as an appetizer.

4   eggs
     Zest of 1 lime
     Juice of ½ lime
2   scallions, thinly sliced
1   6-ounce can crab meat, well rinsed and drained
1   tablespoon fresh chives, chopped
1   Roma tomato, finely diced

Preheat oven to 425°F. Whisk all ingredients together. Fill two 12-hole, nonstick, mini muffin tins 3/4 full with mixture. Bake for 15 minutes or until lightly golden.

ALL PHASES; SERVES 2–4

Sassy Sardine and Egg Spread

This omega-3–rich spread can double as an appetizer when it is stuffed into toma-toes or celery. It might even be served as a light main dish. Kari Wheaton, of Kari's Marvelously Mashed Cauliflower (page 143), says that this spread is terrific with sliced red pepper and cut-up fennel bulb (the vegetable).

1   4-ounce can sardines with bones, drained and flaked
1   tablespoon flaxseed oil
1   tablespoon fresh lemon juice
1   tablespoon apple cider vinegar
1   hard-boiled egg, finely chopped
¼   small onion, finely minced
3   black olives, minced
     Cayenne and dried mustard to taste
     Fresh parsley as garnish

In a medium bowl, combine sardines, flaxseed oil, lemon juice, vinegar, egg, onion, olives, cayenne, and mustard and mash together until well blended. Refrigerate. Serve slightly chilled. Garnish with parsley.

ALL PHASES; SERVES 1–2

Olive Flaxy Spread

This is a quickie spread that makes a terrific snack as a dip for vegetables between meals. It is also an instant topping to finish off grilled chicken, fish, or beef. I personally enjoy this with the Crispy Potato Skins (page 166).

1   cup black olives, rinsed and pitted
1   tablespoon flaxseed oil
1   tablespoon fresh lemon juice
2   small garlic cloves, minced

Place all ingredients in a blender or food processor and chop finely.

Variation:

For phase 3: substitute olive oil for flaxseed oil and add a dash of salt.

ALL PHASES; SERVES 4

Yummy Yam Chips

Whether orange or white, even kids will like these chips.

2   small yams, cut into ⅛-inch slices
½   teaspoon dried basil
½   teaspoon dried oregano
½   teaspoon onion powder

Preheat oven to 300°F. In a self-sealing plastic bag, place yam slices, herbs, and onion powder. Shake to coat. Place the yams on a nonstick baking sheet sprayed with nonstick cooking spray. Bake for about 45 minutes or until yam slices are slightly golden and crispy, making sure to turn at least once during cooking process. Be careful not to burn yam slices.

Variations:
- It is okay to substitute sweet potatoes for the yams. Try changing the flavor mix by substituting sweeter spices such as ground anise and fennel for the Italian herbs. Sprinkle with a dash of cayenne for another kick.
- Substitute ¼ teaspoon cinnamon and 1 packet of Stevia Plus for the Italian herbs for a sweet treat.
- Substitute ¼ teaspoon onion powder, ¼ teaspoon ginger, and ¼ teaspoon cumin for a new savory twist.

For phase 3: sprinkle with salt to taste.

PHASES 2 AND 3; SERVES 2

Pâté for All Seasons

Company's coming. This is a fabulous dip that I first tasted at a Fat Flush party in my home in San Francisco many years ago. My good friend John created it. This is a great party pleaser. It is perfect with veggies or multicolored tortilla chips for phase 3.

2	13-ounce cans water-packed tuna, rinsed and drained
1	8-ounce can oysters, rinsed and drained
1	2-ounce can anchovy fillets, well rinsed and drained
1	garlic clove, minced
2	tablespoons parsley, chopped
1/4	teaspoon dried dill
1/4	teaspoon dried mustard
1	teaspoon fresh lemon juice

Place all ingredients in a food processor or blender and blend until smooth. Add water if needed.

Variation:

For phase 3: add 1/4 teaspoon dried horseradish.

ALL PHASES; SERVES 8

For the Thrill of the Grill

Grilling isn't just for veggies, as you will soon see and savor. Grilled fruits make for interesting appetizers, sensational starters, and succulent tidbits for hors d'oeuvres.

1   apple, cored and cut into rings
    Dash of cloves

Preheat the grill to medium high, coating racks with nonstick cooking spray. Season apple rings with cloves. Place apple rings directly on grill racks turning until fruit is hot and streaked with brown, about 5–7 minutes.

Variations:

- *For phase 1 or 2:* you may replace the apple with a peach or a nectarine.
- For phase 3, you may replace the apple with a pineapple that is cut into rings. Drizzle the rings with a bit of butter seasoned with a dash of dried mint. Same grilling time. Or simply splash some rum over the pineapple before grilling.
- *For phase 3:* you may also try a combo of honeydew and cantaloupe chunks, drizzled with a light butter and mint seasoning, but reduce the grilling time to about 3 minutes.
- *For Special Occasion:* mango and papaya would work very nicely, too. Grilling time with these fruits is about 4 minutes.

ALL PHASES; SERVES 1

Fruity Kebobs

Phase 3 fruits are delicious when grilled, and you can get pretty creative with the combinations. However, be mindful of the portions allowed when you mix and match.

½   banana
½   cup cantaloupe chunks
½   cup pineapple chunks
1   cup strawberries
4   skewers

Preheat the grill to medium high and coat racks with nonstick cooking spray. Make kebabs by alternating banana with cantaloupe, pineapple, and strawberries on the skewers. Place kebabs on the grill rack and cook for about 1½ minutes on each side or until golden.

Variations:
- Substitute a kiwi for the strawberries.
- *For Special Occasion:* try ½ mango instead of the strawberries for a tropical twist. Splash with rum before grilling.

PHASE 3; SERVES 4

Chickpea Pâté

This Mediterranean-style pâté is chock-full of soluble fiber, which is helpful in keeping cholesterol levels low. It tastes great with your favorite veggies or as a salad dressing (just thin it with water) on fresh, leafy greens alongside the Artichoke Frittata (page 69) or on an egg dish of your choice.

1   cup cooked or canned chickpeas (garbanzos), drained, reserving liquid
3   tablespoons onion, chopped
3   tablespoons parsley, chopped
1   garlic clove, minced
1   teaspoon dried basil
½   teaspoon oregano
¼   teaspoon ground cumin
2   tablespoons lemon juice
1   tablespoon liquid from chickpeas

Place all ingredients in a food processor or blender and blend well. Add more liquid if needed.

<small>PHASE 3; SERVES 2</small>

Zesty Avocado Dip

The avocado is a vegetarian source of protein, potassium, and vitamin E. Its high content of the heart-smart monounsaturated omega-9 fatty acids makes this a fruit that's safe to eat. Thinned down with a bit of water to the desired consistency, this zesty dip can double as a salad dressing.

1   small ripe avocado, peeled, pitted, and mashed
¼   cup scallions, finely chopped
¼   cup cilantro, chopped
1   tablespoon lemon juice, freshly squeezed
2   tomatoes, seeded and finely chopped
½   teaspoon ground cumin
½   teaspoon cayenne
1   tablespoon flaxseed oil

Place all ingredients in a large bowl and blend well. Serve with veggies for dipping. Use such veggies as snow peas, jicama, or endive leaves.

Variation:

You may substitute olive oil for the flaxseed oil. Or try adding the seeds of ½ or 1 small pomegranate for a taste treat.

PHASE 3; YIELDS ABOUT 1 CUP

Fat Flush Yogurt Dip

This basic yogurt dip goes well with pungent veggies for dipping, like radishes (especially daikon, which is good for breaking down fat) and yellow, green, and red fresh pepper strips.

1   cup plain, whole milk yogurt
2   tablespoons fresh lemon juice
1/4 cup leek, minced
1   teaspoon dried dill

Combine yogurt, lemon juice, leek, and dill. Chill.

Variations:
- Replace leek with scallions and add 1/2 teaspoon of dried horseradish.
- For a curry-type flavor, replace leek and dill with 1/4 teaspoon ground cumin and 1/4 teaspoon ground turmeric.
- For garlic lovers, replace leek and dill with 2 mashed garlic cloves.

PHASE 3; YIELDS ABOUT 1 CUP

Ranch Style Cottage Cheese Dip

This is an easy-to-assemble dip rich in dairy calcium. Endive leaves and yellow squash rounds make great vegetable dippers.

1   cup low-fat cottage cheese
3   tablespoons fresh lemon juice
1   tablespoon onions, chopped
2   teaspoons fresh parsley, chopped
½   teaspoon garlic powder
½   teaspoon onion powder

Blend all the ingredients in a blender until smooth. Chill at least 1 hour
   before serving.

Variation:

For a Southwestern kick, seed, stem, and chop 1 jalapeño pepper and
¼ cup cilantro into dip.

PHASE 3; YIELDS 1¼ CUPS

Yogurt Cheese

I first learned about this recipe many years ago from my clients in southern California. It is a good, healthy spread (yogurt is filled with beneficial bacteria that aid digestion and protect against pathogens), which is delightful on a slice of toast or simply by itself.

2   cups plain, whole milk yogurt
    Dash of ground nutmeg
    Dash of ground cinnamon
    Dash of ground cardamom

Line a colander with cheesecloth and place colander in a bowl. In another bowl, mix the yogurt with the nutmeg, cinnamon, and cardamom. Pour the yogurt mixture onto the cheesecloth. Place in the fridge, cover, and let drain overnight.

Variation:
Add 1/4 teaspoon vanilla extract for an interesting flavor.

PHASE 3; SERVES 2–4

Fat Flush Nutty Mix

This is a good make-ahead snack when you need some crunch. I personally add a tablespoon or two of this basic mix to plain yogurt or cottage cheese. Nuts are a great source of essential and healthy fatty acids and provide extra vitamin E, fiber, and satiety at snack times.

2   tablespoons butter
1/2   cup almonds
1/2   cup pecans
1/2   cup walnuts
1/2   cup pumpkin seeds
1/4   teaspoon cayenne
1/8   teaspoon ground cinnamon
1/8   teaspoon ground ginger

Melt butter in a medium skillet over medium heat. Add all ingredients to skillet, stirring constantly to blend making sure to coat nuts evenly with spices. Cook until nut mixture is lightly golden brown and toasted, about 6 minutes. Remove from heat and let cool. Store in airtight container.

Variation:

For a Special Occasion: add in 1/4 cup raisins or a mixture of 1/4 cup chopped, dried apricots, dates, or figs.

PHASE 3; SERVES 6

Fat Flush Chickpea Peanuts

These are quite addictive, so be careful on the quantities. This is a great snack for the kids, by the way.

1   can (15-ounce) chickpeas, rinsed well and drained
1   tablespoon sesame oil
¼   teaspoon ground ginger
¼   teaspoon ground coriander
¼   teaspoon ground cumin

Preheat oven to 400°F. In a bowl, mix the chickpeas with the oil and spices. Place on a nonstick baking sheet sprayed with nonstick cooking oil. Bake about 1/2 hour or until chickpeas are golden and crunchy.

Variation:

You may substitute olive oil for sesame oil.

PHASE 3; SERVES 4

Fat Flush Petite Pizza

This easy-to-make, guilt-free pizza snack is surprisingly satisfying and filling.

1   slice Health Seed Spelt, toasted
4   tablespoons no-salt-added tomato sauce
1   ounce mozzarella cheese from part skim milk, grated
     Dash of garlic powder
     Dash of ground fennel
     Dash of dried oregano

Preheat oven to 300°F. Place bread on nonstick cookie sheet. Add oregano to tomato sauce and spread on bread. Sprinkle with garlic powder and fennel. Add cheese. Bake for about 8 minutes or until cheese is melted.

Variation:

Sauté 1/2 cup onions and mushrooms in 2 tablespoons of chicken broth until liquid evaporates and vegetables are caramelized. Add as topping to pizza.

PHASE 3; SERVES 1

Roasted Chestnuts

The most easily digested nuts, chestnuts are really a starchy vegetable. One of my favorite fall and winter snack treats, roasted chestnuts make me think of New York, where vendors sell them on wintry days.

12 chestnuts, rinsed and dried

Preheat oven to 425°F. Cut an X on the side of each chestnut where it is most flat. Place on a nonstick baking sheet in a single layer. Roast in oven for about 20–25 minutes or until chestnuts are tender, turning occasionally. Remove from oven and cool before peeling off the outer and inner shell.

Variation:

Chestnuts go well with a dash of cloves, allspice or nutmeg. They are a nice addition to brown rice as a side dish to an entree.

Phase 3; Serves 3

Shrimp Puffies

These shrimp puffies may seem a bit decadent, but they are delightfully Fat Flush–friendly.

1   egg white
2   tablespoons Spectrum Naturals organic mayonnaise
1   teaspoon garlic powder
½   cup shrimp, cooked and finely chopped
10 large daikon radish rounds

Preheat broiler. In a small bowl, beat egg white until soft peaks form. In another bowl, mix mayonnaise, garlic powder, and shrimp. Fold shrimp mixture into egg white. Place spoonfuls on daikon rounds. Spray nonstick baking sheet with nonstick cooking spray. Broil until golden.

Variation:
Substitute any type of seafood for the shrimp. Lobster, scallops, and crab make good puffies, too.

PHASE 3; SERVES 2

9   Dressings

There is no doubt about it. Dressings can transform simple proteins, salads, veggie side dishes, and fruity desserts into true gourmet delights. You will find flaxseed oil predominating in many of these dressings because it is a staple in all three phases. Just remember it is sensitive to air, heat, and light so try to consume these homemade dressings within a couple of days. Flaxseed oil's nutty flavor is enhanced with aromatic Fat Flush herbs as well as a bit of lemon, lime, and/or apple cider vinegar to aid digestion. Most of these dressings are so easy and fast that you can make them on a daily basis.

By the way, you'll find that mustard is a frequent ingredient in these dressings—not only because of its pungent bite, but because dried mustard has the ability to raise metabolism. (One teaspoon of dried mustard has a 25 percent metabolism-raising effect.)

The Basic Fat Flush
Salad Dressing

Not just for salads, this dressing can be drizzled over steamed veggies. When drizzled over cooked vegetables, the flaxseed oil takes on a buttery taste. (Please see the Fat Flush Vegetable Steaming Guide on pages 128–130 for some varied veggie ideas.)

4   tablespoons flaxseed oil
2   tablespoons apple cider vinegar
2   tablespoons fresh lemon juice
1   teaspoon fresh parsley, chopped

Put all ingredients in a small jar, cover, and shake vigorously until mixed. Use immediately or refrigerate for up to 4 days.

Variations:
- *For phase 1:* Add 1/2 to 1 teaspoon of ground fennel, ground anise, ground coriander, or ground cumin.
- *For phase 2:* Add 1/2 to 1 teaspoon of dried basil, dried oregano, dried mint, or dried rosemary.
- *For phase 3:* Add 1/2 to 1 teaspoon of dried tarragon, dried thyme, or saffron.

ALL PHASES; YIELDS ABOUT 2/3 CUP

Fat Flush Vinaigrette

Here's an idea for a dressing you may want to try when you don't want to use your daily flaxseed for smoothies, let's say, and snacks. This goes well on just about anything green.

5	tablespoons 1-2-3 Chicken Broth (page 222)
1	garlic clove, minced
1	tablespoon apple cider vinegar
1	tablespoon fresh lemon juice
1	tablespoon fresh parsley, chopped
1	teaspoon dried mustard

Put all ingredients in a small jar, cover, and shake vigorously until mixed. Use immediately or refrigerate.

Variations:
- *For phase 1:* Add a few drops of unsweetened cranberry juice concentrate and 1/4 teaspoon Stevia Plus for a cran vinaigrette.
- *For phase 2:* Add 1/2 teaspoon dried basil to seasonings.
- *For phase 3:* Substitute 1 cup of water and 1/4 cup sherry or white wine for the chicken broth, while increasing vinegar to 1/4 cup. Now you have a marinade for chicken, fish, beef, and tofu!

ALL PHASES; YIELDS ABOUT 1/2 CUP

Cilantro-Lime Vinaigrette

This vinaigrette may be used to quickly add zip to any simple tuna, salmon, or shrimp dish. Add more veggies as a side to this dish and you have lunch or dinner in minutes.

½ cup scallions, chopped
2   tablespoons fresh lime juice
2   tablespoons fresh cilantro, chopped
½ teaspoon dried mustard
2   tablespoons flaxseed oil

Combine scallions, lime juice, cilantro, and mustard in a medium bowl. Whisk in flaxseed oil. Use immediately or refrigerate in a small jar for up to 4 days.

ALL PHASES; YIELDS ABOUT ½ CUP

Pass the Flax Dressing

I like this drizzled onto greens—kale, turnip greens, watercress, or escarole.

4   tablespoons of flaxseed oil
3   tablespoons fresh lemon juice
2   garlic cloves, minced
1   teaspoon fresh parsley, chopped
1/2 teaspoon dried mustard

Place all ingredients in a small jar, cover, and shake vigorously until mixed. Use immediately or refrigerate in a small jar for up to 1 week.

Variations:
- Add a grated cucumber, chopped chives, and dash of cayenne for a kick.
- *For phase 3:* turn this into a sautéing liquid by substituting olive oil for the flaxseed oil.

ALL PHASES; YIELDS ABOUT 1/2 CUP

Fat Flush French Dressing

Here's a dressing you can prepare several days ahead of time. The Fat Flush Catsup (page 206) is an integral ingredient in this dressing. Please keep this dressing refrigerated after you use it because of the fragility of flaxseed oil. This is a perfect fancy dressing for company. Try drizzling it over plain old baked chicken or fish for an epicurean delight.

1   cup flaxseed oil
½   cup Fat Flush Catsup
1   teaspoon Stevia Plus
⅓   cup apple cider vinegar
½   teaspoon dried mustard
2   garlic cloves, minced

Place all ingredients in a blender and mix well. Transfer to a small covered jar and use immediately or store in the fridge for up to 1 week.

ALL PHASES; YIELDS ABOUT 1¾ CUP

Emerald Greens Dressing

This is great with leafy greens, chopped fresh veggies, or any of the Fat Flush seafood entrees.

4   tablespoons of flaxseed oil
1   tablespoon apple cider vinegar
4   tablespoons green pepper, chopped
½   teaspoon dried dill
1   tablespoon fresh parsley, chopped
1   tablespoon onion, chopped

Place all ingredients in a small jar and shake vigorously until mixed. Use immediately or store in the fridge for up to 4 days.

ALL PHASES; YIELDS ABOUT ⅔ CUP

Creamy Lemon-Lime Yogurt Dressing

Using yogurt instead of flaxseed, olive, sesame, or grape seed oil in dressings allows you to use these flavorful oils instead for drizzling or cooking. The Creamy Lemon-Lime Yogurt Dressing goes well with the Creamy Lemon-Lime Crab Salad (page 68).

1   cup plain, whole milk yogurt
1   tablespoon fresh lemon juice
1   tablespoon fresh lime juice
½   teaspoon dried mustard
1   small onion, grated
1   teaspoon dried basil
⅛   teaspoon cayenne
1   garlic clove, minced

Combine all ingredients in bowl. Cover and refrigerate for at least 30 minutes before using. May be stored in fridge for up to 1 week.

PHASE 3; YIELDS ABOUT 1¼ CUPS

Nutty Avocado Dressing

Avocados, with their buttery smooth consistency, make delicious dressings for both vegetable salads and fruit salads. Here I have added some omega-3 rich crunch with the pumpkin seeds and the toasted wheat germ. The avocado picks up the flavor of the foods it is combined with.

2	ripe avocados, peeled, pitted, and mashed
4	tablespoons toasted pumpkin seeds, chopped
3	tablespoons toasted wheat germ
2	tablespoons lime juice

Mix all ingredients together in a small bowl until well blended. Use immediately or store in fridge for up to 4 days.

PHASE 3; YIELDS 1½ CUPS

Garlicky Avocado Dressing

This makes a great accompaniment to Warm Thai Lamb Salad (page 71).

2 small avocados, peeled, pitted, and mashed
2 garlic cloves, minced
4 tablespoons fresh lemon juice
4 tablespoons flaxseed oil

Mix all ingredients together in a bowl until well combined. Use immediately or store in fridge for up to 4 days.

PHASE 3; YIELDS 1½ CUPS

Cinnamon Yogurt Dressing

This is a great dress-up for simple fruit desserts. Why not enjoy it over Saucy Rhubarb (page 249), Baked Cranberry Apples (page 250), or Spiced Vanilla Peaches (page 256)?

1   cup plain, whole milk yogurt
½   teaspoon vanilla extract
1   teaspoon Stevia Plus
     Lemon zest
¼   teaspoon ground cinnamon
     Pinch of ground nutmeg

Mix all ingredients together in a bowl and chill. Store in fridge for up to 1 week.

PHASE 3; YIELDS ABOUT 1 CUP

California Guacamole Dressing

I especially like this over main dish salads featuring shrimp, crab, or scallops. It also makes a great dip.

1   avocado, sliced
1/2   red onion, sliced
1   tablespoon fresh lemon juice
1   tablespoon fresh cilantro, chopped
1   garlic clove, minced
2   tablespoons grape seed oil or olive oil
2   tablespoons apple cider vinegar
1½   tomato, chopped

Place all ingredients, except 1/2 chopped tomato, in a blender and blend until smooth. Pour into a small bowl and mix in remaining chopped tomato.

PHASE 3; YIELDS ABOUT 1 CUP

Minty Sesame Dressing

This is a great, nutty-flavored dressing to drizzle on steamed broccoli, cauliflower, cabbage, or string beans (pages 128–130). The Minty Sesame Dressing is a perfect accompaniment to the Lamb Salad with Mint (page 72).

¼　cup sesame oil
3　tablespoons fresh lemon juice
2　tablespoons onion, chopped
1　teaspoon toasted sesame seeds
1　teaspoon fresh mint, chopped

Place all ingredients in a blender. Blend until smooth.

Variations:
- Try substituting olive oil for the sesame oil.
- Use toasted pumpkin seeds instead of the sesame seeds.

PHASE 3; YIELDS ¼ CUP

10 Condiments, Sauces, and Such

Condiments represent the spice of life and are perfect toppings, coatings, seasonings, accompaniments, and spreads for Fat Flush breakfast foods, entrées, veggies, snacks, and sweet indulgences. The original Fat Flush Catsup and the newly created Cran-Jewel Catsup are good on absolutely everything. I guess you can say that's also true of the salsas, sauces, and pestos.

Adding these unusual condiments to your meals, as you probably know by now, isn't just for taste appeal but for health. I am sure you will want to try your own hand at being creative with these various condiments. For example, you can roll and coat all kinds of Fat Flush fruits and veggies, with the Omega-rich toasted and ground flaxseeds for a heart-smart, fiber-filled crust. You can also dress up veggies (eggplant, squash, okra) and fish, poultry, beef, and tofu with the flax and Fat Flush Bread Crumbs.

I think that you will find that even a single addition of one of the condiments can perk up a meal. I personally enjoy the Fat Flush Curry Seasoning or West Indian Seasoning when I need a zesty lift for my dips and sauces. I especially like the Minty Dill Pesto on plain tuna or salmon when I don't have time to fuss.

If you make up condiments ahead of time, you can always use them as easy snacks between meals. Between lunch and dinner, I typically grab a handful of nuts (though not until Phase 3) to keep me going before supper and have even been known to relish the Home Made Salsa as a between-meal pick-me-up.

Toasted Flaxseeds

Toasted and ground flaxseeds are a perfect Fat Flush accompaniment to yogurt, cottage and ricotta cheeses, cereal, and salads and are a crunchy coating for cut-up fruit!

Remember: You are allowed 2 tablespoons per day of ground flaxseeds. If you choose to use the Toasted Flaxseeds as a topping or coating for foods, these will still count as your 2 tablespoons per day of flaxseed fiber and so, accordingly, eliminate flaxseed from the Long Life Cocktail (and if you are using the psyllium, eliminate it there as well).

1   cup whole flaxseeds

Preheat oven to 250°F. Spread flaxseeds on a baking sheet and place in oven. Bake for 15–20 minutes until crispy. Grind in a flaxseed or coffee grinder. Store in fridge or freezer.

Variations:
- For all phases, you may season with a dash of onion powder, garlic powder, and cayenne, the Fat Flush Curry Seasoning (page 204). Or you may blend cloves, cinnamon, and anise for a sweeter touch.
- *For phase 2:* add a dash of dried basil to the flaxseeds.
- *For phase 3:* try some ground cardamom.

ALL PHASES; YIELDS ABOUT 1 CUP

Toasted Nuts or Seeds

Crunchy, flavorful, and high in the amazing omegas, nuts and seeds can encrust fish and chicken as well as add some fiber to vegetables, yogurt, dips, cottage cheese, and salads. Here's the best way to prepare them for good digestion and good taste.

1   cup nuts or seeds (raw almonds, filberts, pecans, peanuts, pistachios, macadamia nuts, pumpkin seeds, sunflower seeds)

Preheat oven to 250°F. Spread raw nuts or seeds on baking sheet. Place in oven and bake for about 15–20 minutes or until golden. Store in fridge or freezer.

PHASE 3; YIELDS 1 CUP

Storage Tip: Nuts and seeds last longer when they are stored in the fridge or in a dry, cool place away from light. They can also be stored in the freezer for about a year in an airtight container.

Fat Flush Bread Crumbs

Bread crumbs work well as fillers or coatings for entrées. Here's the Fat Flush way to make bread crumbs. Hint: stale bread will produce drier bread crumbs.

2   slices Health Seed Spelt bread, toasted and cooled

Place slices of bread in blender or food processor. Process until bread resembles fine bread crumbs.

Variations:
- *For phase 2:* add a pinch of dried oregano and dried basil per 1/4 cup of breadcrumbs.
- *For phase 3:* add 2 tablespoons of grated Parmesan cheese.

PHASES 2 AND 3; YIELDS 1/2 CUP

Fat Flush Curry Seasoning

Here's a tasty and creative way to blend the flavor factors of the thermogenic spices with their fat-burning powers. The Fat Flush Curry Seasoning is great for waking up veggies and simply broiled chicken, fish, and seafood.

4   tablespoons ground coriander
1   tablespoon ground cumin
1   tablespoon dried fennel
1   tablespoon cayenne
1   tablespoon ground cinnamon
1½ teaspoons ground turmeric
5   whole cloves

Crush all the ingredients together using a mortar and pestle or grind together in a food processor until fine. Store in an airtight container in the refrigerator or in a cool, dry place away from heat and moisture.

Variation:
For phase 3: add 3 ground cardamom seeds to the mix for extra flavor.

ALL PHASES; YIELDS APPROXIMATELY ½ CUP

Fat Flush West Indian Seasoning

Here's a variation of the mixes popular in the islands of the West Indies. This rendition really spices up seafood, meats of all kinds, and poultry. You can be as creative as you like according to your taste preferences. This one is a bit hot. You can make this fresh weekly and change the ingredients for more or less heat.

4   scallions, chopped
½   cup lime juice, fresh
½   cup fresh parsley, chopped finely
1   garlic clove, minced
2   small jalapeños, seeded and minced
1   teaspoon cayenne

Place all ingredients in a food processor or blender. Process until finely chopped. Transfer to a storage container. Cover and refrigerate.

Variations:
• *For phase 2:* Add 1 teaspoon dried rosemary.
• *For phase 3:* add 2 teaspoons of dried thyme to the original recipe and enjoy.

ALL PHASES; YIELDS ABOUT 1 CUP

Fat Flush Catsup

This recipe, which first appeared in The Fat Flush Plan, is not just for grown-ups. My nephews use this catsup on almost everything—from scrambled eggs to burgers to meatloaf and veggies such as carrots and broccoli. It is a primary ingredient in the Fat Flush French Dressing (page 190) and Fat Flush Cocktail Sauce (page 206).

2   tablespoons Muir Glen Tomato Purée
1½ teaspoons apple cider vinegar
⅛   teaspoon Stevia Plus
½   teaspoon garlic, finely minced
     Pinch of cayenne

Place all ingredients in a small bowl and whisk until well blended. Keep refrigerated.

ALL PHASES; SERVES 1

Fat Flush Cocktail Sauce

This is a nice way to dress up seafood appetizers. The Fat Flush Catsup (see above) plays an important part in this saucy blend.

2   tablespoons Fat Flush Catsup
1   teaspoon fresh lemon or lime juice
¼   teaspoon dried mustard
1   teaspoon fresh cilantro, finely chopped
3   pinches cayenne, to taste

Prepare the Fat Flush Catsup as directed. Add the lemon (or lime) juice, mustard, cilantro, and cayenne. Whisk until well blended.

ALL PHASES; SERVES 1

Homemade Salsa

I like this with cut up jicama, snow peas, and cucumber. In phase 3, of course, a handful of corn chips hits the spot. The Homemade Salsa is lovely with the Artichoke Frittata (page 69).

1–2   fresh, small jalapeños, minced (optional)
⅛   cup fresh cilantro, finely minced
¼   cup green pepper, finely minced
2   garlic cloves, finely minced
1   14.5-ounce can no-salt-added Muir Glen Diced Tomatoes, drained
     Juice of ½ lime
6   scallions (white parts only), finely diced
2   tablespoons apple cider vinegar

In a medium bowl, mix all ingredients until well blended. Refrigerate a few hours or overnight.

ALL PHASES; YIELDS ABOUT 2 CUPS

Pico de Gallo Sauce

A main ingredient in Pico de Gallo Eggs (page 55), this serves up nicely as a condiment for grilled beef and broiled fish.

1½ pounds fresh tomatoes, seeded and finely chopped
1   large red onion, finely chopped
2   jalapenos, seeded and minced (optional)
¼   cup fresh cilantro, chopped
3   tablespoons fresh lime juice
4   tablespoons 1-2-3 Chicken Broth (page 221)

In a small bowl, mix all ingredients until well blended. Cover and let sit
    for at least 1 hour before serving.

ALL PHASES; YIELDS ABOUT 1 CUP

Cran-Jewel Catsup

This mix goes well with everything just like the regular catsup. Especially good with leftover turkey or chicken, try this out on your burgers as well.

½   pound cranberries, fresh or frozen thawed
      Seeds of ½ pomegranate
½   cup red onion, thinly sliced
½   cup purified water
¼   cup apple cider vinegar
1   teaspoon Stevia Plus
¼   teaspoon ground cloves
¼   teaspoon ground cinnamon

In a medium saucepan over medium heat, cook the cranberries, pomegranate seeds, onion, and water until cranberries soften. Stir constantly to avoid burning. Place cranberry mixture into a food processor or blender and blend until smooth. Place the mixture back into the saucepan. Add vinegar, Stevia Plus, cloves, and cinnamon to the mixture. Stirring constantly, cook until thickened, approximately 8–10 minutes. Keeps well in the fridge.

Variation:
In phase 3: 1/4 teaspoon of salt may be added.

ALL PHASES; YIELDS ABOUT 1 CUP

Hearty Barbecue Sauce

This is a terrific addition to Stuffed Onion Casserole (page 80) and is also good for basting plain meats, poultry, and fish on the grill or in the oven.

½   cup onion, finely chopped

2   garlic cloves, minced

2   tablespoons plus ¼ cup 1-2-3 Beef Broth (page 223), divided

¼   cup apple cider vinegar

1   teaspoon onion powder

½   teaspoon Stevia Plus

1   8-ounce can no-salt-added Muir Glen Tomato Purée

1   teaspoon cayenne, or to taste

½   jalapeño, seeded and minced

Sauté onion and garlic in 2 tablespoons broth until tender. Add remaining broth, vinegar, onion powder, Stevia Plus, tomato purée, cayenne, and jalapeño. Bring to a boil, reduce heat, and simmer for about 30 minutes. Cool and store in the fridge.

ALL PHASES; YIELDS ABOUT 1 CUP

Special Occasion Instant Spice Rub

No time to make a roast taste special? Use this molasses-based spice rub on a 4–5 pound pot roast or lamb roast for a guaranteed pleasing taste. And this mix really gives baked beans a memorable tang.

2   tablespoons olive or grape seed oil
1   tablespoon molasses
1¼ teaspoons cayenne
½   teaspoon dried mustard
¼   teaspoon onion powder
¼   teaspoon garlic powder

In a bowl, mix all ingredients. Spread evenly over the roast or blend well into baked beans.

PHASE 3 SPECIAL OCCASION; YIELDS ABOUT 3 TABLESPOONS

Quick Cran-Raspberry Sauce

This seems like such a natural for Fat Flush French Toast (page 62), especially when you have no time to cook. It is also tasty in yogurt in phase 3.

½   cup cranberries, fresh or frozen thawed
½   cup raspberries
½   teaspoon orange zest
¾   teaspoon Stevia Plus

Place all ingredients in a blender and blend until smooth. Heat in a saucepan for about 2 minutes or until hot.

ALL PHASES; SERVES 1

Greek Tszitziki Sauce

This sauce may easily double as a snack. I especially enjoy it with a steamed arti-choke (page 127) or over a chopped parsley, olives, onions, and tomato salad.

½   cucumber, peeled, seeded, and diced
1   cup plain, whole milk yogurt
1   tablespoon fresh parsley, chopped
1   tablespoon fresh dill or basil, chopped

Place all ingredients in a small bowl, mix well, cover, and chill for 3–4
   hours before serving.

Variation:

Try adding ½ teaspoon dried oregano with the parsley and dill or basil.

PHASE 3; YIELDS ABOUT 1½ CUPS

Minty Dill Pesto

Rather than an ordinary pesto, why not try a pesto made the Fat Flush way? The three herbs I have combined here offer a new flavor experience. In this recipe, the fresh dill, mint, and basil are much more flavorful than the dried herbs. This is divine on any kind of white fish (cod, sole, haddock, or halibut), and I personally enjoy spooning this onto fresh green vegetables, especially broccoli and kale. The Minty Dill Pesto goes well with Salmon Cakes (page 87).

2   tablespoons walnuts, chopped
2   garlic cloves, minced
2   tablespoons fresh dill, chopped
1   tablespoon fresh mint, chopped
2   tablespoons fresh basil, chopped
4   tablespoons flaxseed oil

Place all ingredients in a blender or food processor and blend until puréed.

PHASE 3; SERVES 4

Basil Pesto

This classic dressing enhances just about everything it touches. I love it the best on a medley of colorful and fresh vegetables. It's a good way to get the kids to eat their veggies.

¼   cup fresh basil, chopped
⅛   cup grated Parmesan cheese
⅛   cup flaxseed oil
2   garlic cloves, minced
⅛   cup pine nuts
⅛   cup olive oil

Place all ingredients in a blender and blend until smooth.

PHASE 3; SERVES 4

Clove-Scented Flaxseed Oil

Somehow the nutty, buttery flavor of flaxseed oil lends itself best to sweeter, more aromatic spices. This blend is grand over steamed yellow squash and spaghetti squash.

4   tablespoons flaxseed oil
     Dash of ground cloves

In a small bowl, blend together flaxseed oil and cloves. Use immediately.

Variation:

For phases 2 and 3: Try this drizzled over baked sweet potato, yam, or acorn squash.

ALL PHASES; YIELDS 4 TABLESPOONS

Cinnamon-Scented Flaxseed Oil

This blend goes best drizzled over a baked apple.

4   tablespoons flaxseed oil
    Dash of cinnamon

In a small bowl, blend together flaxseed oil and cinnamon. Use immediately.

Variations:
- *For phases 2 and 3:* Drizzle over toasted Ezekiel 4:9 or HealthSeed Spelt.
- *For Special Occasion:* Toss a few raisins into the blend and drizzle over ricotta cheese sweetened with 1/4 teaspoon of Stevia Plus.

ALL PHASES; YIELDS 4 TABLESPOONS

Flaxy Butter Spread

Here's the perfect margarine substitute for your whole family. This is a flavorful flax-butter that is especially good for adding to veggies after they are cooked and for smearing on Ezekiel 4:9 toast. Compound butters like this stay fresh in the fridge for up to 2 weeks or in the freezer for up to 1 month.

½ cup (1 stick) butter, softened to room temperature and cubed
½ cup of flaxseed oil

In a saucepan on low heat, place butter cubes until they lightly melt. Transfer melted butter to a storage container, adding flaxseed oil and blending well. Cover and store in fridge or freezer until spread solidifies.

Variation:
Add a dash of cinnamon for a sweet taste or a dash of cayenne for a spicy flavor.

PHASE 3; YIELDS ABOUT 1 CUP

Dilled Butter Spread

Here's a variation on the flaxy spread theme—but this time without the flax! This spread is delicious spread on scrambled or hard-boiled eggs and is wonderful with fish, especially salmon.

½ cup (1 stick) butter, softened to room temperature
½ cup fresh dill, chopped, or about ⅛ cup dried and crushed dill

In a small bowl, blend together butter and dill until creamy and smooth. Cover and chill for a couple of hours to bring out the flavor.

PHASE 3; YIELDS ABOUT 1 CUP

French Butter Spread

I love this spread with all kinds of vegetables, especially asparagus and broccoli. My clients say that it is delightful smeared on toasted HealthSeed Spelt.

½   cup (1 stick) unsalted butter, softened to room temperature
1   tablespoon fresh parsley, chopped
1   teaspoon dried and crushed chives
1   teaspoon dried and crushed tarragon

In a small bowl, blend together butter and herbs until smooth and creamy. Cover, refrigerate, and serve chilled.

Variation:

Try replacing the parsley, chives, and tarragon with 2 teaspoons of dried and crushed mint and 1 teaspoon of dried and crushed anise. Serve melted on steamed peas.

PHASE 3; YIELDS ½ CUP

Cilantro Butter Spread

½   cup (1 stick) unsalted butter, softened to room temperature
½   cup fresh cilantro, chopped
1   garlic clove, minced
1   teaspoon fresh lime juice

In a small bowl, blend together butter, herbs, and lime juice until smooth and creamy. Cover, refrigerate, and serve chilled.

PHASE 3; YIELDS ABOUT 1 CUP

Flaxy Syrup

When you need a sweet topping, this one comes in handy, especially for the kids. This is made to go with Fat Flush French Toast (page 62) in place of the cranraspberry sauce.

4   tablespoons maple syrup
4   tablespoons flaxseed oil

Blend together and store in fridge.

Variation:

Adding spices like ground cloves, anise, cinnamon, or nutmeg can hit the spot.

PHASE 3 SPECIAL OCCASION; SERVES 4

11 Stocks and Soups

Soup is a wonderful way to get in your veggies. The Fat Flush broths that were featured in *The Fat Flush Plan* are so essential to phases 1 and 2 cooking that they are repeated here for your convenience. As many Fat Flushers already know, the broths are a marvelous substitute for oils and poaching liquids, they keep foods moist, and they pick up the delicate tastes of herbs and spices. I always use the 1-2-3 Chicken Broth recipe instead of water for imparting a unique flavor to brown rice, for example, in phase 3.

Insider Tip: You may want to freeze broths in an ice cube tray for convenience; 1 tablespoon of broth is equivalent to one 1 cube of broth. Frozen stock should keep in the freezer for up to about 3 months.

Insider Tip: Use cold water for making a soup—especially the broths. This allows the nutrients from the chicken and chicken pieces or beef and bones to absorb into the soup rather than be sealed into the meat and bones.

Insider Tip: Cool soup before placing it into the fridge. This saves wear and tear on the refrigerator motor, which can work overtime to cool down extra-hot foods that are placed in the fridge.

Insider Tip: If soup is frozen, first thaw it out to room temperature and then reheat it. This preserves the flavor.

Insider Tip: Soup is a great way to fill yourself up before going out to a party or special occasion, where you just know you will be tempted with non-Fat Flush foods.

EASY SOUPS

BASIC BROTHS

1-2-3 Vegetable Broth

This will come in handy all by itself as a soup or as cooking stock for other dishes.

2   quarts purified water
1   large onion, cut into 1-inch pieces
3   celery stalks, cut into 1-inch pieces
1   carrot, cut into 1-inch pieces
1   bunch scallions, chopped
8   garlic cloves, minced
8   sprigs fresh parsley
8   ounces mushrooms cut in ½-inch slices
2   bay leaves

Place all ingredients in a large stockpot and bring to a boil. Reduce heat and simmer uncovered for about 1 hour. Strain and discard vegetables and bay leaves. Refrigerate and use within 3 days, or freeze.

Variation:

For phase 2 or 3: You may sweeten the pot by adding 1 small sweet potato, cubed.

ALL PHASES; SERVES 4

1-2-3 Chicken Broth

*This broth is delicious as a clear soup all by itself as a meal starter or as a snack.
This broth can be used as a cooking stock for other dishes. To remove any fat, chill
broth and skim off fat, which will rise to the top.*

2   quarts purified water
3   pounds chicken pieces with bones
3   tablespoons apple cider vinegar
1   large onion, cut into 1-inch pieces
3   celery stalks, cut into 1-inch pieces
1   carrot, cut in 1-inch pieces
4   sprigs parsley
2   bay leaves

Place all ingredients in a large pot and bring to a boil. Reduce heat, cover,
and simmer for about 45 minutes or until the chicken is done. Strain
and discard vegetables, bones, and bay leaves and save the chicken
for another dish. Refrigerate and use within 3 days, or freeze.

Variations:
- *For phase 2 or 3:* Add 1 small sweet potato, cubed, to the pot.
- To make a rich, brown sauce, leave onion skin on.

ALL PHASES; SERVES 4

1-2-3 Beef Broth

Similar to the vegetable and chicken broths, this broth can be used for sautéing other foods or by itself as a light soup. To remove any fat, chill broth and skim off fat, which will rise to the top.

3   pounds beef shank bones
1   large onion, cut into 1-inch pieces
2   quarts purified water
3   tablespoons apple cider vinegar
3   celery stalks, cut into 1-inch pieces
1   carrot, cut into 1-inch pieces
4   sprigs fresh parsley
4   garlic cloves, minced
2   bay leaves

Preheat oven to 450°F. Place bones and onion in a roasting pan. Bake for 30 minutes or until bones are browned. Remove from oven.

Place bones and onion in a large stockpot. Add water, vinegar, celery, carrot, parsley, garlic, and bay leaves to the stockpot and bring to a boil. Reduce heat, cover, and simmer for 3 hours. Strain and discard vegetables and bones and save the meat for later use or another recipe. Refrigerate and use within 3 days, or freeze.

Variations:
- *For phase 2 or 3:* Add 1 small sweet potato, cubed.
- To make a rich, brown sauce, leave onion skin on.

ALL PHASES; SERVES 4

EASY SOUPS

Soups are a perfect candidate for a quick meal because they can be made ahead and frozen. With the exception of the Gingery Egg Drop Soup and Purée of Asparagus Soup that are best fresh, all the soups here can be made ahead and frozen.

When it comes to freezing soups, first let the soup cool to room temperature and then freeze it in jars or containers, making sure to leave a couple of inches at the top because the liquid will expand when frozen. Also, seal tightly so the soups do not lose their flavor.

Gingery Egg Drop Soup

There are many variations to this satisfying soup. You can use chopped cilantro or parsley to replace the scallions.

½   teaspoon fresh gingerroot, grated
1   cup no-salt-added chicken broth or 1-2-3 Chicken Broth (page 222)
1   egg, beaten
2   tablespoons scallions, chopped

In a medium saucepan, add grated gingerroot to chicken broth and bring to a boil. Reduce heat to simmer. Pour the egg into the broth slowly, stirring constantly to create egg shreds. Garnish with scallions.

ALL PHASES; SERVES 1

Purée of Asparagus Soup

Many vegetables can be used with this puréed soup. Look at our variations below.

1 pound asparagus spears, trimmed and blanched
½ cup plus 2½ cups 1-2-3 Vegetable Broth (page 223), divided.
¼ onion, chopped
1 garlic clove, chopped
   Pinch of dried mustard
   Lemon zest, to taste

In a large saucepan, sauté asparagus, onion, and garlic in ½ cup broth until onions are tender. Transfer the mixture to a food processor or blender. Add remaining broth and purée until smooth. Pour into a pot and simmer, covered for 20 minutes. Add mustard and lemon zest. Serve immediately.

Variations:
- Substitute yellow squash for the asparagus and substitute a pinch of aromatic cloves and fennel for the mustard.
- Substitute cauliflower for the asparagus and substitute a pinch of cumin for the mustard to provide an earthy flavor.
- Substitute celery for the asparagus and omit the mustard and lemon zest.

ALL PHASES; SERVES 4

Rose's Fat Flush Soup

This is a tasty Fat Flush standby created by Rose Grandy, "Lady Rose" on the Fat Flush Messaging Board. Many Fat Flushers have used this meal-in-a-soup to keep themselves fueled up and filled up throughout the day.

1	pound ground beef or turkey
16	ounces Muir Glen Tomato Purée
16	ounces purified water
½	onion, chopped
1	cup spinach
1	cup green beans, chopped
2	garlic cloves, minced
½	medium green pepper, chopped
½	medium red pepper, chopped
1	celery stalk, chopped
1	bay leaf
1	tablespoon fresh parsley, chopped

Brown the meat in a skillet over medium heat until it is no longer pink. Drain fat. Place the browned meat with all other ingredients in a large pot. Cook over low-medium heat for about 1 hour. Remove the bay leaf and serve hot.

Variation:

Substitute cooked, diced chicken for the beef.

ALL PHASES; SERVES 4

Very Veggie Soup

Did you know that carrots, celery, and parsley are considered higher-sodium vegetables? They impart a naturally salty (and satisfying) flavor to this soup, without any added salt. Along with potassium, sodium is required for the proper functioning of our nerves and the contraction of our muscles (like the heart, our hardest-working muscle). Fluid balance, electrolyte balance, and pH (acid/alkaline) balance depend upon sodium.

2   cups 1-2-3 Vegetable Broth (page 221)
1   zucchini, sliced
2   carrots, sliced
1   celery stalk, sliced
½   tablespoon fresh parsley or coriander for garnish

Combine all ingredients in a medium-sized pot. Bring to a boil. Reduce heat, cover, and simmer for 20 minutes or until vegetables are tender. Purée soup in a blender. Garnish with fresh parsley or coriander.

Variation:

For a chunkier texture, omit the puréeing.

All Phases; Serves 2

Hot and Sour Shrimp and Vegetable Soup

This is an all-in-one meal when you don't have time for side dishes.

5   cups no-salt-added chicken broth or 1-2-3 Chicken Broth (page 222)
1/4   cup apple cider vinegar
1/2   teaspoon Stevia Plus
1/4   teaspoon cayenne
1/4   teaspoon ground ginger
1   pound raw shrimp, peeled and deveined
1 1/2 cups radishes, sliced
1 1/2 cups spinach, shredded
2/3   cup scallions, sliced
1   cup Enoki mushrooms for garnish (optional)

Bring broth to a boil in a large soup pot. Stir in vinegar, Stevia Plus, cayenne, and ginger. Add shrimp and cook until shrimp turn pink and curl, about 3–4 minutes. Remove from the heat. Stir in radishes, spinach, and scallions. Cover and let stand 2–3 minutes before serving. Garnish with Enoki mushrooms, if desired.

ALL PHASES; SERVES 4

Gazpacho

This is a cold soup favorite that even the kids will like. Notice that flaxseed oil is used instead of the more traditional olive oil to make this an omega-3 winner.

4	tomatoes, peeled, seeded, and coarsely chopped
1/2	cup onion, chopped
1/2	cucumber, peeled, seeded, and chopped
1/2	green pepper, seeded and chopped
1	garlic clove, minced
2	tablespoons flaxseed oil
3	tablespoons apple cider vinegar
1/2	cup cold purified water
2	tablespoons fresh parsley

Place all ingredients in a blender or food processor. Blend until smooth. Serve in chilled bowls.

Variation:

For phase 3: Top with a dollop of sour cream or plain yogurt.

ALL PHASES; SERVES 4

Creamy Mushroom Soup

Mushrooms are a source of energy-producing B vitamins and immune-boosting zinc. They also contain glutamic acid, another source of energy. The presence of tofu provides a creamy consistency.

1   pound button mushrooms, thinly sliced
    Pinch of cumin
1   teaspoon onion powder
1   tablespoon plus 2 cups 1-2-3 Chicken Broth (page 222), divided
2   teaspoons plus 3 tablespoons lemon juice, divided
1   bunch watercress, chopped
½   cup onion, chopped
1½ cups silken tofu
2   tablespoons fresh parsley or cilantro or combination, chopped

In a medium saucepan over medium heat, steam mushrooms, cumin, onion powder, 1 tablespoon of the broth, and 2 teaspoons of the lemon juice. Steam for about 10 minutes, stirring occasionally. Drain steamed mixture and set aside, reserving the liquid in the pot.

To the pot, add the watercress and chopped onion. Sauté for 2 minutes. Add remaining broth and ½ of the mushroom mixture and simmer for another 10 minutes. In a blender, place mixture, tofu, parsley (or parsley/cilantro combination), and the remaining lemon juice and purée. Place the purée mixture back in the pot, add the remaining mushrooms, reheat, and serve.

ALL PHASES; SERVES 4

Creamy Red Pepper Soup

Red pepper is a great source of vitamin C and provides a touch of natural sweetness to this soup.

1   large red pepper, chopped
2   small leeks (white part only), chopped
½   cup onion, chopped
2   teaspoons fresh dill
½   teaspoon chives
¼   teaspoon onion powder
3   tablespoons plus 2 cups 1-2-3 Chicken Broth (page 222), divided
3   tablespoons fresh cilantro, chopped
1   cup silken tofu

Combine red pepper, leeks, onion, dill, chives, onion powder, and 3 tablespoons of the chicken broth in a medium size pot. Sauté over medium heat for 8 to 10 minutes or until tender, adding more broth if needed. Add remaining broth, bring to a boil, lower heat, and simmer for 20 minutes. Remove from heat and let stand for 10 minutes. After cooled, purée in blender with cilantro and tofu. Return to pot and warm before serving.

ALL PHASES; SERVES 2

Green Dream Soup

This really tastes good, even if you are not a Brussels sprouts fan!

1	pound Brussels sprouts, trimmed
	Purified water
1/4	teaspoon cinnamon
	Juice of 1/2 lemon
	Handful of fresh cilantro
2	cups 1-2-3 Chicken Broth (page 222)

Place Brussels sprouts in saucepan and cover with 4 inches of water. Bring to a boil, reduce heat to medium, and cook for 10 minutes covered. Drain Brussels sprouts, reserving liquid. Set liquid aside. Place Brussels sprouts and remaining ingredients in a blender. Purée until smooth. If too thick, add some of reserved liquid until desired consistency is obtained. Serve warm.

ALL PHASES; SERVES 2

Spinach Soup

4   scallions, chopped
2   garlic cloves, minced
4   cups spinach, well packed
¼   cup plus 2 cups 1-2-3 Vegetable Broth (page 221)
1   bay leaf
1   teaspoon onion powder
1   tablespoon fresh parsley or cilantro
1   12-ounce package of tofu
    Juice of ½ lemon
    Juice of ½ lime

In a large saucepan over medium heat, cook scallions and garlic in ¼ cup of broth for 8 minutes or until soft. Stir in the spinach, cover, and cook for additional 5 minutes. Add the remaining broth, bay leaf, and onion powder. Simmer in covered saucepan for an additional 5 minutes. Remove the bay leaf. Purée the soup in blender, adding parsley or cilantro, tofu, and lemon and lime juice. Reheat if needed and serve immediately.

ALL PHASES; SERVES 4

Tofu Shrimp Soup

A meal in one, like Rose's Fat Flush Soup, this soup is very filling and nourishing.

1   tablespoon fresh ginger, chopped
3   garlic cloves, minced
2   tablespoons plus 4 cups 1-2-3 Chicken Broth (page 222), divided
1   cup carrots, sliced
1   cup broccoli florets
1   cup water chestnuts, sliced
1   cup mushrooms, sliced
½   cup bamboo shoots, sliced
2   tablespoons apple cider vinegar
1   pound firm tofu, cut into 1-inch cubes
1   pound shrimp, peeled and deveined
2   cups mustard greens, cut roughly
¼   cup parsley, chopped
2   tablespoons scallions, chopped

In a large pot, sauté ginger and garlic in 2 tablespoons of broth for 2 minutes. Add remaining broth, carrots, broccoli, water chestnuts, mushrooms, bamboo shoots, and vinegar and bring to a boil. Cook until crisp-tender. Add tofu and shrimp. Reduce heat and simmer until shrimp is cooked, about 3–5 minutes. Add mustard greens, cooking until greens are lightly cooked but still crisp. Sprinkle the soup with parsley and scallions. Serve right away or freeze.

ALL PHASES; SERVES 4

Velvety Avocado Soup

This is a delightful cold soup for hot summer days. I like this as a breakfast soup.

1   cup 1-2-3 Chicken Broth (page 222)
½   avocado, peeled and sliced
1   apple (Golden Delicious), peeled, cored, and sliced
½   cup plain whole milk yogurt
     Juice of 1 lime
     Parsley for garnish

In a saucepan, heat broth and set aside. Place avocado, apple, yogurt, and lime juice in blender and blend until creamy. Blend in broth. Serve at room temperature or chilled. Garnish with parsley.

PHASE 3; SERVES 1

CHAPTER

12   Beverages

There are many creative and secret ways (without cheating!) to adapt the Fat Flush principles to healthy and thirst-quenching beverages. Certain herbal teas, as you will discover in this section, can be made from the Fat Flushing herbs and spices allowed in each phase. These special teas do not take the place, of course, of the recommended cran-water, lemon and water, or plain water in the daily three-phase protocols, but they can be used as delightfully fragrant and satisfying additions—about 1 to 2 cups per day, if you wish, between meals and snacks.

Homemade Cranberry Juice

Unsweetened cranberry juice is such a major Fat Flush staple that I wanted to reprint this recipe from The Fat Flush Plan. *This is a tried-and-true recipe for making your own unsweetened cranberry juice for the cran-water component of the program in phase 1 and for the Long Life Cocktail components in phases 2 and 3. Although Stevia Plus is suggested as a sweetener (if you can't take it straight), I much prefer that you develop a taste for the tart but oh-so-smart cranberry without any sweetening because it is this very tart taste that opens up the liver's detoxification pathways. By the way, cranberries are no longer seasonal fruits available only at Thanksgiving and Christmas. Stahlbush Farms carries organic frozen cranberries all year round.*

1   12-ounce bag cranberries, frozen or fresh
4   cups purified water
    Stevia Plus to taste (optional)

Place cranberries and water into a large saucepan. Boil until berries pop. Strain the juice and refrigerate. Add Stevia Plus to taste.

ALL PHASES; YIELDS ABOUT 32 OUNCES

Cinnamon-Cranberry Tea

Rose Grandy created this unusual beverage. Simply subtract this ¼ cup (or 2 ounces) of unsweetened cranberry juice from your daily allotment and you have Cinnamon Cranberry Tea.

¼ cup unsweetened cranberry juice
¾ cup purified water
½ teaspoon ground cinnamon

Combine cranberry juice and water in a small saucepan. Bring to a quick boil. Reduce heat and stir in cinnamon. Serve warm.

ALL PHASES; SERVES 1

Fat Flush Lemonade

On a warm summer day, there is nothing like real lemonade. Here is the Fat Flush version that you can enjoy and even serve to your company. The lemonade should take the place of the hot water and lemon in all three phases and can be enjoyed twice a day as a treat.

¼ cup lemon juice, freshly squeezed
¼ teaspoon Stevia Plus or to taste
2   cups chilled, purified water

Combine all ingredients until the Stevia Plus is completely dissolved. Serve chilled.

Variations:
- ¹/4 cup freshly squeezed lime juice can be substituted for the lemon juice.
- ¹/4 cup unsweetened cranberry juice can be substituted for the lemon or lime juice for a cranade.

ALL PHASES; SERVES 2

Gingerroot Tea

Gingerroot tea is warming and can help digestion if it is taken with a meal. It helps regulate the system, aids in controlling diarrhea and stomach cramps, and tastes good as well. A bit of Stevia Plus may be used for sweetening.

1   teaspoon fresh gingerroot
1   pint purified water

Place the gingerroot in the water in a small saucepan. Boil for about 15–20 minutes. Remove from heat, strain, and enjoy hot or cold.

Variations:

- Journalist Marlene Martin, who writes for *The Light Connection* and interviewed me about *The Fat Flush Plan*, suggests adding a cinnamon stick to the pot and boiling it along with the gingerroot for a delightful and aromatic cinnamony flavor. She also is fond of a pinch of ground anise and ground cloves in her gingerroot tea.
- If you feel a cold coming on, add a dash of cayenne, 1 large clove of minced garlic, and the juice of half a lemon to your tea.
- *Phase 3 Special Occasion:* You can even add 1 teaspoon of honey.

ALL PHASES; SERVES 1

Fennel Tea

Fennel is an excellent herb for relieving gas and indigestion. Used by mothers for years to control infant colic, the licoricelike taste lends itself well to teas for adults.

1   teaspoon whole fennel seeds
1   pint purified water

Place the seeds in the water in a small saucepan. Boil for about 15–20 minutes. Strain and enjoy hot or cold.

ALL PHASES; SERVES 1

Parsley Tea

Parsley is a great natural diuretic, high in potassium and other alkalinizing minerals. This tea is very helpful for relief of painful urination.

1   teaspoon fresh parsley
1   pint purified water

Place the parsley in the water in a small saucepan. Bring to a simmer for about 15 minutes. Strain and enjoy, hot or cold.

ALL PHASES; SERVES 1

Spiced Dandylion

This recipe is a wonderful way to spice up your beverages with a little kick from ginger, cinnamon, and cloves.

1   cup brewed dandelion root coffee
¼   teaspoon ginger
½   teaspoon cinnamon
    pinch of cloves
1   cup purified water

Combine all ingredients in a large mug and enjoy!

ALL PHASES; SERVES 2

Peppermint Tea

Very refreshing, peppermint tea is cleansing of and calming to the nervous system.

1   teaspoon fresh peppermint (spearmint can also be used as a substitute)
1   pint purified water

Place the peppermint in the water in a small saucepan. Bring to a simmer for about 15 minutes. Strain and enjoy, hot or cold.

PHASES 2 AND 3; SERVES 1

Hot Cocoa

Bet you thought you'd never see this one in a Fat Flush cookbook. The cream is very satisfying and actually quite good for the nervous system.

1   rounded tablespoon cocoa powder
1½ teaspoons vanilla extract
¼   teaspoon Stevia Plus
¾   cup purified water
¼   cup cream

Combine all ingredients in a small saucepan. Whisk together until the cocoa is blended. Heat until just simmering. Serve hot.

Enjoy!

PHASE 3 SPECIAL OCCASION; SERVES 1

Hot Carob

If you are allergic to cocoa or want to avoid it because of its high copper content, why not try carob?

1   rounded tablespoon carob
1½ teaspoons vanilla
¼   teaspoon Stevia Plus
¾   cup purified water
¼   cup cream

Combine all ingredients in a small saucepan. Whisk together until the carob is blended. Heat until just simmering. Serve hot.

PHASE 3 SPECIAL OCCASION; SERVES 1

13 Nourishing Sweets and Indulgences

Naturally, the best desserts of all are those that Mother Nature provides.

However, you will be impressed that the treats in this section make it so easy to get the sugar out and still satisfy anybody's sweet tooth on Fat Flush. Whether as a dessert or a snack, you will be pleasantly surprised at how satisfying these naturally sweetened recipes really are. Cinnamon is used frequently in these easy desserts, because it helps to regulate blood sugar levels. Many of the desserts, like Cinnamony Apple Sauce and the Fat Flush Cheesecake, use the sweetener Stevia Plus, made from the herb stevia from South America. As many of you already know from *The Fat Flush Plan*, stevia does not raise blood sugar or create yeast problems.

For special occasions or for a healthful dessert option for the family, you will find that some recipes in this section do use minimal amounts of more traditional sweeteners. For instance, unsweetened fruit juices are used in the Blueberry Pecan, Strawberry Almond, and Tropical Paradise Jells, date sugar in the Apple Crisp, and honey in the Lemony Almond Cookies. The fruity jells and other treats are great healthy desserts for the kids anytime and for you too when you feel like having a comfort food. (Just keep in mind that if you are strictly following the Fat Flushing Food Combination Rules from *The Fat Flush Plan*, you will want to separate your main meal from your dessert by at least an hour to optimize digestion.)

What you won't see in this section are any desserts made with fructose—a sweetener that is ranked the lowest on the glycemic index. The glycemic index is a listing of foods that shows the rate at which a carbohydrate breaks down as sugar or glucose into the bloodstream. Although fructose lends itself well to desserts and a little goes a long way (it is one and a half times sweeter than ordinary sugar or sucrose), fructose has many health drawbacks. It can increase artery clogging LDL-cholesterol levels, raise uric acid levels in the blood, and raise triglyceride levels more than any other type of sugar. The fructose that naturally occurs in fruits, however, is combined with both fiber and minerals which balance out fructose's negative health effects when it is consumed only as an isolated sweetener.

Before we begin, please keep in mind that many of the desserts herein contain meringue (stiffly beaten egg whites) so following are just a few pointers from the get go to get you in the meringue mood. These pointers will greatly help you to get the meringues to hold their shape:

- When the recipe calls for egg whites, you will be making meringues out of them.
- Take the eggs out of the fridge at least 1/2 hour before you start. Egg whites at room temperature produce a fluffier and faster whip than do cold eggs whites.
- The best kinds of bowls to use for making meringues are glass or metal.
- The frothiness or volume of the meringue may be reduced if the bowls are not clean, so take a damp cloth with a bit of apple cider vinegar and wipe them thoroughly to cut any residue.
- You will know when the meringues are ready when the egg whites become shiny and do not slip and slide in your bowl.
- To test if your meringues are at their peak (no pun intended), try turning the bowl upside down. If the meringues cling to the bowl, they are ready for prime time.
- Cream of tartar is a marvelous meringue stabilizer and is good for you, too. Cream of tartar is made from grapes, is a decent source of potassium, and, according, to folk medicine, is a natural blood cleanser. This ingredient fits the Fat Flush criteria, now doesn't it?
- Make sure you watch the meringues carefully because they can burn easily. Go for a lightly golden color.
- Do keep in mind that meringues made without sugar are not as crispy as those made with sugar—the Fat Flush–style meringues will not have the same texture as those made with sugar.

Cinnamony Applesauce

This aromatic applesauce recipe lends itself to many varieties of apples such as the ones listed below. You may also use Golden Delicious, Jonathan, Pippin, or Winesap. I like Cinnamony Applesauce after one of the poultry entrées, especially Dijon Turkey Cutlets (page 105) or Crispy Nonfried Chicken (page 107).

1   apple (Rome Beauty, Granny Smith, or McIntosh), peeled, cored, and sliced
¼   teaspoon Stevia Plus or to taste (optional)
½   teaspoon cinnamon

Preheat oven to 300°F. Arrange apple slices in a small baking dish. Sprinkle with Stevia Plus and cinnamon and cover. Bake for 15 minutes. Mash when cooked and serve hot or cold.

Variations:
- For a change of pace, substitute cherries (omit the cinnamon), berries, or a peach for the apple.
- Try a touch (just a touch) of cloves.
- *For phase 3:* Add a drop of vanilla extract and a dash of allspice and nutmeg.

ALL PHASES; SERVES 1

Saucy Rhubarb

Whether warmed or slightly chilled, cooked rhubarb with a bit of Stevia Plus is a nice alternative to applesauce. One cup of this unique fruit has more calcium (350 mg) than a cup of milk. This recipe goes well with Zucchini and Beef Delight (page 116).

1   pound rhubarb, chopped
1   tablespoon purified water
4   teaspoons Stevia Plus
1/2 teaspoon cinnamon

In a medium saucepan, cook rhubarb in water over low to medium heat 12–15 minutes. Mash and blend in Stevia Plus and cinnamon.

Variations:
- Add a cup or two of strawberries or the seeds of 1/2 of a small pomegranate, which seems to go so well with rhubarb.
- *For phase 3:* Sprinkle with 2 tablespoons of chopped walnuts, pecans, or almonds to add some crunch and omega-3 power.

ALL PHASES; SERVES 4

Baked Cranberry Apples

Here's your basic baked apple recipe with some uniquely Fat Flush–friendly fillings.

4   medium apples (Rome Beauty, McIntosh, Golden Delicious), cored and pared
½   cup cranberries, fresh or frozen (thawed)
1   teaspoon Flora-Key or Stevia Plus
1   teaspoon cinnamon
3–4 tablespoons purified water

Preheat oven to 350°F. In a small bowl, blend cranberries, Flora-Key or Stevia Plus, and cinnamon. Stuff apples with cranberry mixture. Place in shallow baking dish, add water in the baking dish with the fruit and cover. Baste fruit with liquid during cooking and bake for about 30–40 minutes.

Variations:
- Chopped walnuts or pecans, grated lemon or orange zest, nutmeg, cloves, or allspice are tasty phase 3 variations as well.
- *For Special Occasion:* Top with a tablespoon of homemade whipped cream.
- *For phase 3–Special Occasion:* you can transform this recipe into Baked Cranberry Raisin Apples by adding 1 tablespoon of raisins to each apple and a dash of nutmeg, too.

ALL PHASES; SERVES 4

Tofruity Freeze

This is a surefire way to get used to the taste of soy for those twice-a-week soy fests (you remember, of course, from The Fat Flush Plan *that soy is recommended twice a week.) The good thing about this dessert is that the soy-based tofu provides you with some protein, natural fats, and natural phytohormones, which is why Tofruity Freeze makes a good snack.*

1   10.5-ounce package silken tofu
2   cups berries, fresh or unsweetened frozen

Put tofu in the blender and blend until it attains a puddinglike consistency. Add fruit and continue to blend until smooth. Pour into freezer containers or ice-cube trays. Freeze for several hours until lightly firm.

Variations:
- You may substitute the right amount of cherries for the berries and add a touch of Flora-Key or Stevia Plus if the fruit is not sweet enough.
- *For phase 3:* Top with toasted sunflower seeds and/or 1 tablespoon of unsweetened coconut.

ALL PHASES; SERVES 2

Pomegranate Ice

Did you know that the very first sherbet on record was made with snow and pomegranate juice? If you have been good and do not have blood sugar peaks and valleys, there is no reason why you shouldn't treat yourself to this puréed fruit dessert. Just remember that puréeing breaks down the fiber in fruits, which can have a fluctuating effect on blood sugar by concentrating the sugars. If this makes you hungry, you can always pop in 1 package of silken tofu to provide some blood sugar–stabilizing protein and fat.

    Seeds of ½ or 1 small pomegranate
1   teaspoon fresh lemon juice
¼–½   teaspoon Flora-Key or Stevia Plus (optional, to taste if fruit is not sweet enough)

To remove the seeds from pomegranate, cut the rind into quarters and pull apart in a bowl of water, removing seeds from membrane. Remove the membrane and the rind with a slotted spoon. Place strainer in large bowl and pour into strainer to drain and recover seeds. Place all ingredients in a food processor or blender and purée until smooth. Freeze until firm, about 3–4 hours.

Variation:
A blend of 1 cup raspberries and strawberries can replace the pomegranate.

ALL PHASES; SERVES 1

Cranberry Mousse

This is so easy to make and quite lovely as a tangy refreshment to complete a cozy brunch or dinner.

2   cups cranberries, fresh or frozen (thawed)
1½ cups purified water
     Juice of 1 lemon
1   teaspoon lemon zest
2   teaspoons Flora-Key or Stevia Plus (more or less to taste)
2   egg whites, stiffly beaten, with pinch of cream of tartar

In a medium saucepan, combine cranberries and water and cook until soft. Strain and discard skins. Add lemon juice, lemon zest, and Flora-Key or Stevia Plus to strained cranberries. Pour into freezer containers or ice-cube trays. Freeze about 3–4 hours until frozen. When frozen, remove from freezer, beat until mixture is softened. Fold in egg whites. Pour into freezer containers or ice cube trays. Return to freezer and freeze until ready to serve.

Variations:

• Replace one or both cups of the cranberries with pomegranate seeds.
• *For phase 3:* sprinkle with slivered almonds and 1 tablespoon of unsweetened coconut.

ALL PHASES; SERVES 4

Blueberry Mousse

You really can enjoy some treats on phases 1 and 2. This Blueberry Mousse proves it.

1   cup blueberries
1   teaspoon Flora-Key or Stevia Plus (or to taste)
1   egg white
    Pinch of cream of tartar

Place blueberries and Flora-Key or Stevia Plus in blender and purée until smooth. Beat egg white with cream of tartar until stiff peaks form. Stir in 1/4 of egg white into blueberry mixture to "lighten." Gently fold in remaining egg whites. Pour into a small freezer container with lid and freeze until firm. Partially defrost for 10 minutes and serve.

Variation:
Add 1 block whipped silken tofu for an extra-creamy treat.

ALL PHASES; SERVES 1

Vanilla Fat Flush Ice Cream

You won't believe this until you try it. For those of you who have that ice cream urge, here's a healthy way to satisfy the urge without all that sugar. Whey protein powders sweetened with stevia actually become sweeter when frozen—and they come in many different legal Fat Flush flavors. That's the secret in this quick and easy rendition.

1   scoop vanilla-flavored whey-based protein powder
1/4 cup cold purified water

In a small bowl, blend whey powder and water. Pour into a freezer container and freeze until ready to serve.

Variation:
Top with a sprinkling of toasted ground or milled flaxseeds.

ALL PHASES; SERVES 1

Strawberry Fat Flush Ice Cream

This is so easy, it's a sin.

1   scoop strawberry-flavored whey-based protein powder
¼   cup cold purified water

In a small bowl, blend whey powder and water. Pour into a freezer container and freeze until ready to serve.

Variation:
Top with a sprinkling of toasted ground or milled flaxseeds.

ALL PHASES; SERVES 1

Chocolate Fat Flush Ice Cream

If you think that the Vanilla and Strawberry Fat Flush ice creams (page 254 and above) were good, this is the best tasting yet.

1   scoop chocolate-flavored whey-based protein powder
¼   cup purified cold water

In a small bowl, blend whey powder and water. Pour into a freezer container and freeze until ready to serve.

Variations:
- Piña-colada–flavored whey-based protein powder and tropical-twist-flavored whey-based protein powder can alternate with the chocolate in phase 3 and for special occasions.
- Top with 1 teaspoon of toasted walnuts and shredded, unsweetened coconut.

PHASE 3; SERVES 1

Spiced Vanilla Peaches

This is a personal, all-time favorite.

4   peaches, peeled, cored, and halved
1   tablespoon purified water
1   teaspoon allspice
12 drops vanilla extract

Preheat oven to 350°F. Place peaches and water in baking dish. Sprinkle
with allspice and drizzle each peach half with 3 drops of vanilla
extract. Cover and bake for about 20 minutes. Serve warm.

Variations:

- Fresh plums, nectarines, Bartlett pears, and apples may be substituted
  for the peaches, and any of these are also delightful with a dash of allspice and a touch of vanilla.
- Serve with Marinated Shrimp Over Squash (page 90) for a gourmet
  ending to a flavorful meal.

PHASE 3; SERVES 4

Peachy Keen Sorbet

This is a lovely light dessert after a meal of beef, veal, or lamb that is surprisingly satisfying without the sugar.

4   peaches, peeled, cored, and cubed
2   teaspoons almond extract
1   teaspoon Flora-Key or Stevia Plus
1/2 teaspoon fresh lemon juice

Place all ingredients in a blender or food processor and blend until smooth. Freeze in plastic containers or ice-cube trays for about 2 hours. Take out partially frozen fruit and stir well to break up ice crystals. Return to freezer and freeze completely. Let stand at room temperature 15 minutes before serving.

Variation:

This sorbet can be made with other types of fruit and flavorings. Try substituting pears for the peaches and adding 1/4 teaspoon of powdered gingerroot.

PHASE 3; SERVES 4

Razzle Dazzle Sorbet

The special ingredient in this sorbet is bananas. They give this dessert a consistency almost like ice cream. Do note that this sorbet provides 1½ fruit servings per person, so adjust additional fruit intake accordingly.

2 cups raspberries (fresh or frozen)
2 bananas, sliced
1 teaspoon Flora-Key or Stevia Plus
½ teaspoon fresh lemon juice

Place all ingredients in a blender or food processor and blend until
smooth. Place in a plastic containers or ice-cube trays and freeze at
least 2 hours. Take out partially frozen mixture and stir well to break
up ice crystals. Return to freezer to freeze completely. Let sorbet stand
15 minutes at room temperature before serving.

Variations:

- Any type of berry can be used in place of the raspberries. Blueberries
  are especially good and very high in a health-promoting and brain-
  boosting substance called anthocyanins—an antioxidant belonging to
  the flavonoid family.
- *For phase 3 Special Occasion:* Substitute 1 tablespoon honey for the Stevia Plus.

PHASE 3; SERVES 4

Grape Sorbet

Grapes are delightful—especially when they are transformed into this sorbet, which is so simple and surprisingly satisfying.

12 large grapes

1/2 teaspoon lemon juice

1/4 teaspoon Flora-Key or Stevia Plus (optional to taste if fruit is not sweet enough)

Fresh mint leaf for garnish

Place all ingredients in a food processor or blender and purée until smooth. Place in a plastic container and freeze at least 2 hours. Take out partially frozen mixture and stir well to break up ice crystals. Return to freezer to freeze completely. Let stand at least 15 minutes before serving. Garnish with mint.

Variation:

For a Special Occasion: try 1/2 mango or 1/3 medium papaya for a tropical twist topped with toasted macadamias and unsweetened shredded coconut.

PHASE 3; SERVES 1

Berry Yogurt Freezes

Taste what a touch of yogurt can do! The kids will really enjoy these treats. They won't even know that they are healthy.

2   cups berries (strawberries, raspberries, or blueberries)
4   tablespoons plain whole milk yogurt
1/4 to 1/2 teaspoon Flora-Key or Stevia Plus (optional to taste if fruit is not sweet enough)

Place berries, yogurt, and Flora-Key or Stevia Plus in blender and blend until smooth. Pour into popsicle molds or small paper cups with popsicle sticks and freeze until solid.

Variations:
- For a Not Just Berry Yogurt Freeze, substitute 2 peaches for a flavor twist.
- Top with 2 tablespoons of coconut, toasted almonds, or toasted sunflower seeds.

PHASE 3; SERVES 2

Strawberry-Banana Freeze

If Berry Yogurt Freezes (see page 260) are for kids, then Strawberry-Banana Freeze definitely has "grown-up" written all over it. This is simple and fast. (Don't forget that ½ banana is one fruit exchange, so, with this treat, you will be using all of your fruit allotments.)

½   banana
1   cup strawberries
1   cup plain, whole milk yogurt
¼   to ½ teaspoon Flora-Key or Stevia Plus (optional to taste if fruit is
     not sweet enough)
     Dash of cardamom

Place all ingredients except cardamom in a food processor or blender and
      purée until smooth. Pour into ice-cube trays and freeze until solid (at
      least 3 hours). Serve frozen with a dash of cardamon.

Variation:
Top with toasted, chopped walnuts.

PHASE 3; SERVES 1

Fat Flush Cheesecake

Deprive yourself no more! This simple but luscious cheesecake was created by Ellen Buier, who added bananas to give it that creamy texture we adore. With the Quick Cran-Raspberry Sauce (page 211), this is simply divine.

1   pound 2 percent cottage cheese
1   cup mashed ripe banana
2   packets Stevia Plus
    Juice of 1 lemon
4   eggs, beaten
½   teaspoon vanilla extract

Preheat oven to 350°F. Place cottage cheese in a blender and blend until smooth. Add mashed banana, lemon juice, and Stevia Plus and blend until mixed. Beat eggs one at a time and add to the mixture, blending well after each addition. Stir in vanilla extract. Pour the mixture into a lightly greased (use butter), 8-inch springform cake pan. Bake for 35 minutes. Remove from oven and loosen cake from sides of pan with a knife. Cool and then chill for several hours or overnight before serving.

Variation:

Add a splash of rum before pouring mixture into cake pan for baking.

PHASE 3; SERVES 8

Crustless Custard-Pumpkin Pie

Yes, Virginia, there is a Fat Flush style pumpkin pie. High in beta-carotene, this pumpkin pie is sweetened with honey, molasses, and Stevia Plus. With the traditional pumpkin pie spices of ginger, nutmeg and cloves, your family or guests may not even know this dessert is 100 percent sugar-free! Serve with Roast Turkey with Lemon, Garlic, and Fennel (page 103).

1 15-ounce can pumpkin
2 tablespoons honey
2 teaspoons molasses
1 teaspoon cinnamon
1 egg yolk
⅛ teaspoon ginger
⅛ teaspoon nutmeg
¼ teaspoon cloves
¼ teaspoon Stevia Plus
2 egg whites
 Pinch of cream of tartar

Preheat oven to 350°F. In a bowl, thoroughly blend together all ingredients except the egg whites and cream of tartar. Place egg whites in a large bowl, add cream of tartar, and beat until they form soft peaks. Fold the pumpkin mixture into the egg whites and pour into a lightly greased (use butter), 9-inch pie plate. Bake for 45 minutes to 1 hour or until toothpick comes out clean. Cool before serving.

Variation:

For phase 3 Special Occasion: Top with homemade whipped cream, sweetened with Stevia Plus if desired.

PHASE 3 SPECIAL OCCASION; SERVES 8

Blueberry Pecan Jell

This basic gelatin recipe can be made with any type of unsweetened fruit juice. I use the seaweed gelatin agar-agar in my gelatin desserts because it is vegetarian; provides magnesium, calcium, and fiber; and soothes and lubricates the intestinal tract by absorbing moisture. Agar-agar is available in health food stores.

2   cups Mountain Sun blueberry juice or unsweetened fruit juice of choice
4   tablespoons toasted pecans, chopped
½   teaspoon agar-agar

Combine juice, nuts, and agar-agar in saucepan, heat to boiling, stirring constantly. Boil for 30 seconds and remove from heat. Pour into sherbet glasses. Cool for about 20 minutes and refrigerate until set (about 2 hours). Serve chilled.

PHASE 3 SPECIAL OCCASION; SERVES 4

Strawberry Almond Jell

2   cups Mountain Sun strawberry juice or unsweetened fruit juice of choice
4   tablespoons toasted almonds, chopped
½   teaspoon agar-agar

Combine juice, nuts, and agar-agar in saucepan, heat to boiling, stirring constantly. Boil for 30 seconds and remove from heat. Pour into sherbet glasses. Cool for about 20 minutes and refrigerate until set (about 2 hours).

PHASE 3 SPECIAL OCCASION; SERVES 4

Black Cherry Walnut Jell

2 cups Knudsen black cherry juice or unsweetened fruit juice of choice
4 tablespoons toasted walnuts, chopped
½ teaspoon agar-agar

Combine juice, nuts, and agar-agar in saucepan, heat to boiling, stirring constantly. Boil for 30 seconds and remove from heat. Pour into sherbet glasses. Cool for about 20 minutes and refrigerate until set (about 2 hours).

PHASE 3 SPECIAL OCCASION; SERVES 4

Apple Cranberry Sunflower Jell

2 cups Knudsen apple cranberry juice or unsweetened fruit juice of choice
4 tablespoons toasted sunflower seeds
½ teaspoon agar-agar

Combine juice, seeds, and agar-agar in saucepan, heat to boiling, stirring constantly. Boil for 30 seconds and remove from heat. Pour into sherbet glasses. Cool for about 20 minutes and refrigerate until set (about 2 hours).

PHASE 3 SPECIAL OCCASION; SERVES 4

Tropical Paradise Jell

2   cups Mountain Sun Tropical Punch (mixture of unsweetened
    pineapple, grape, mango, and papaya juices) or unsweetened fruit
    juice of choice
½   teaspoon agar-agar

Combine juice and agar-agar in saucepan, heat to boiling, stirring constantly. Boil for 30 seconds and remove from heat. Pour into sherbet
glasses. Cool for about 20 minutes and refrigerate until set (about 2
hours).

PHASE 3 SPECIAL OCCASION; SERVES 4

Frozen Berry Mousse

2   cups strawberries (or berries of your choice)
¼   cup unsweetened apple juice
2   egg whites
    Pinch of cream of tartar

In a blender or food processor, purée berries with the apple juice. Transfer
purée to a bowl. In another bowl, beat the egg whites with the cream
of tartar until egg whites form soft peaks. Fold into purée mixture,
blending well. Freeze until firm around edges, then stir once again
and place back in freezer until firm throughout.

Variation:

Instead of strawberries, try blueberries with 1 teaspoon of lemon zest.

PHASE 3 SPECIAL OCCASION; SERVES 4

Cherry Soufflé

48 cherries, fresh or frozen (thawed)

3 tablespoons honey (or Stevia Plus to taste)

1 tablespoon fresh lemon juice

5 egg whites

Pinch of cream of tartar

Preheat oven to 300°F. In a blender or food processor, purée the cherries. In a medium saucepan, combine the purée and honey. Over low heat, cook approximately 20 minutes or until mixture thickens. Add lemon juice and let mixture sit until lukewarm. In a large bowl, beat egg whites with the cream of tartar until soft peaks form. Carefully fold eggs whites into cherries. Spoon mixture into ungreased soufflé dish. Place soufflé dish in pan of hot water, bake for 1 hour or until soufflé is firm and lightly browned.

(Note: Soufflé can fall if oven door opens before end of baking period.)

PHASE 3 SPECIAL OCCASION; SERVES 4

Apple Crisp

The oat flour in this recipe is especially light and sweet. Healthier than wheat flour, oat flour is lower on the glycemic index than regular flour. If you can't find oat flour in your health food store or grocery, you can always make it at home by grinding rolled oats in your food processor until you get a flour consistency. This crisp is good hot or cold and is a perfect accompaniment to just about any Fat Flush entrée.

⅔   cup date sugar
½   cup oat flour
½   cup old-fashioned rolled oats
⅓   cup butter, softened
1   teaspoon cinnamon
1   teaspoon nutmeg
3   medium apples (Granny Smith, Golden Delicious, or Rome Beauty), cored, peeled, and sliced

Preheat oven to 375°F. In a bowl, mix date sugar, flour, oats, butter, cinnamon, and nutmeg together. Add the apple slices and toss lightly. Pour into 8-inch-square, nonstick baking pan. Bake for about 30 minutes or until apples are soft.

Variations:
• Add a cup of cooked cranberries for added color and antioxidant power.
• Top with 4 tablespoons of raisins.

PHASE 3 SPECIAL OCCASION; SERVES 4

Lemony Almond Cookies

These are flourless cookies made with ground almonds. They are a bit soft right out of the oven, but they harden up when cooled down. These are best stored in an air-tight container.

2   egg whites
    Pinch of cream of tartar
2   tablespoons honey
½   teaspoon vanilla extract
1   tablespoon lemon zest
1   cup almonds, ground

Preheat oven to 250°F. Beat egg whites with the cream of tartar until stiff white peaks form, gradually beating in honey, vanilla, and lemon zest. Gently fold in almonds. Drop 1 tablespoonful of batter at a time on a nonstick or lightly greased (use butter) regular cookie sheet, spacing about 2 inches apart. Bake for about 30 minutes.

Variation:

Try roasted, ground pumpkin seed instead of the almonds and omit the lemon zest.

PHASE 3 SPECIAL OCCASION; YIELDS ABOUT 1 DOZEN COOKIES

Almond Oats Macaroons

The addition of the almond butter adds protein power, B vitamins, potassium, magnesium, calcium, and vitamin E. The healthy fat content of the almond butter also provides satiety, so you should be satisfied with just a couple.

2   egg whites
    Pinch of cream of tartar
1   ounce honey
¼   teaspoon ground cinnamon
½   ounce almond butter
2½ ounces old-fashioned rolled oats

Preheat oven to 275°F. In a large bowl, beat egg whites with cream of tartar until stiff peaks form. Add honey, cinnamon, and nut butter, and continue beating until mixed. Fold in the rolled oats. Drop 1 teaspoonful at a time onto a nonstick or lightly greased (use butter) regular cookie sheet. Bake for 20–25 minutes.

PHASE 3 SPECIAL OCCASION; YIELDS 20

Parsnip Dream

A most unusual dessert, Parsnip Dream was a favorite of my late mentor, Dr. Hazel Parcells. When frozen, parsnips become sweeter. (They also provide fiber, vitamins A and C, potassium, calcium, and beautifying silica.)

2   cups frozen parsnips (previously cleaned and frozen whole)
1   pint heavy cream
2   teaspoons honey
½   teaspoon vanilla extract
¼   teaspoon ground cardamom
8   toasted walnut pieces (for garnish)

Grate frozen parsnips into a bowl and set aside. In another bowl, whip cream until it is very stiff. Add honey, vanilla, and cardamom to the cream and whip until mixed. Fold grated parsnips into the cream. Pour into 4 individual serving glasses. Top with walnuts. Chill.

PHASE 3 SPECIAL OCCASION; SERVES 4

My Mother's Meringue Kisses

Ever since I was a little girl, I enjoyed these melt-in-your-mouth cookie fluffs. Of course, in those days my mother didn't know that sugar was bad (and neither did I). And, I tried and tried with my test kitchen to get these to work with Stevia Plus. No luck. So here are those meringue kisses from yesteryear updated to Fat Flush standards but, alas, you will have to delay your reward for phase 3 Lifestyle.

4   egg whites
¼   teaspoon cream of tartar
1   tablespoon honey
1   teaspoon vanilla extract

Preheat oven to 250°F. As you beat egg whites, add cream of tartar. Combine the honey and vanilla, adding to egg whites as whites begin to stiffen and form soft peaks. Spray a cookie sheet with nonstick cooking spray. Place 8 meringue mounds on cookie sheet and make indentations with back of a spoon. Bake in oven for about 1¼ hours or until meringues become crispy. Turn off oven but let meringues remain in oven to cool. When crispy, remove from oven and store in covered container.

Variation:

Turn the kisses into meringue nests by topping with some Quick Cran-Raspberry Sauce (page 211). Serve by filling with toasted, chopped pecans (or any toasted nut or seed of your choice) and unsweetened coconut shreds.

PHASE 3 SPECIAL OCCASION; YIELDS 8

Surprise Sorbet

The surprise ingredient in this unusual dessert is . . . onions. Onions? Yup. They are great when prepared this way. A friend shared this recipe with me several years ago, and I changed some of the ingredients to make it Fat Flush friendly and fabulous.

2   small onions, finely chopped
1   small scallion, finely chopped
1   tablespoon maple syrup
1   tablespoon apple cider vinegar
⅛   teaspoon cinnamon
⅛   teaspoon cloves
½   cup plain whole milk yogurt

Steam onions until translucent and purée in food processor or blender. In a bowl, combine scallion, maple syrup, vinegar, cinnamon, and cloves. Add puréed onion. Place in glass bowl, cover, and freeze until gently firm. Take out of freezer and blend until sorbet-type consistency. Mix in yogurt and put back in freezer. Serve cold.

PHASE 3 SPECIAL OCCASION; SERVES 1

14 Resources and Support

WWW.ANNLOUISE.COM

This is the best place on the Web to check into regarding all kinds of Fat Flush updates. You will find a store that is well stocked with all the products that have the Fat Flush seal of approval. My calendar is updated regularly on the site regarding my media events, lectures, and radio or TV appearances.

You can also go to www.ivillage.com/diet/fatflush.

And of course, on www.annlouise.com you are most cordially invited to become part of The Forum, an interactive messaging board for further support, ideas, and sharing of your results every day of the week, 365 days a year. There are five outstanding veteran Fat Flush community leaders who are in constant touch with me. On our Forum, you will get your Fat Flush questions answered, and you will be the first to know the latest Fat Flush updates. Our community is dedicated to making your Fat Flush journey a rewarding and healthful experience. On the Forum, there is a special section devoted to Fat Flush cooking and recipes. You can post your Fat Flush creations and share some scrumptious ideas with Fat Flushers all over the world.

FAT FLUSH PRODUCTS AND EDUCATIONAL RESOURCES

Uni Key Health Systems

P.O. Box 2287
Hayden Lake, ID 83835
208-762-6833
Fax: 208-762-9395
Toll free: 800-888-4353
Web: *www.unikeyhealth.com*
Email: unikey@unikeyhealth.com

Uni Key Health Systems is the official distributor of all my products, books, and services. Uni Key carries the Royal Prestige Cookware, the MAC knives, the ultimate flax seed grinder, Doulton ceramic water filters, as well as many of the specialty Fat Flush supplements, including the popular Fat Flush Kit. Uni Key also carries high lignan flaxseed oil, flaxseed oil capsules, Flora-Key, Stevia Plus, dandelion root tea and the Fat Flush Whey.

French Meadow Bakery

2610 Lyndale Ave. South
Minneapolis, MN 55408
877-669-3278; 877-NO-YEAST
www.frenchmeadow.com

This company offers the very best tasting and nutritious organic breads that are dairy-free, yeast-free, oil-free, and sugar-free. The Fat Flush Tortillas and the Healthseed Spelt bread featured in phases 2 and 3 of Fat Flush are made by this company. The spelt bread is high in protein and fiber and is made with flax, pumpkin, and sunflower seeds as well as sprouted legumes and grains. French Meadow has also ventured into functional foods in the form of Women's Bread and Men's Bread.

nSpired Natural Foods

14855 Wicks Boulevard
San Leandro, CA 94577
www.nspiredfoods.com/pmpkrnmn.html
510-686-0116; Fax: 510-686-0126

nSpired Natural Foods is the manufacturer of Pumpkorn, a delicious high-zinc snack food made of pumpkin seeds. If you can't find this product locally, you may call or visit the company's Web site and order the product directly.

FAT FLUSH FRIENDS ON THE WEB

www.expertfoods.com
888-621-9059

This company has some very innovative low-carb products made from vegetable gums. Its Thicken Thin line seems to have the most promise for Fat Flush. I have been looking for a Fat Flush–friendly substitute for cornstarch for the longest time, and its ThickenThin not/Starch thickener seemed to work pretty well for sauces, stews, creamed soups, and even scrambled eggs.

www.aboutproduce.com

This site is sponsored by the Produce for Better Health Foundation. It provides great information about produce in general—what health values certain fruits and veggies contain, how to eat in season, and what the best availability dates are for produce. The nutrition dictionary and recipe search engine are good as well.

www.5aday.com

The National Cancer Institute sponsors this site, which contains helpful information that will empower your consumption of fruits and veggies on Fat Flush.

www.flaxcouncil.ca

This site contains some very interesting flax info, and you can find some great flax recipes which I am sure you can convert to Fat Flush specifications.

www.fatsforhealth.com

This is a comprehensive online guide for essential fatty acid (EFA) information and news. You can get up-to-date data, articles, and news about EFAs in health, nutrition, beauty, disease treatment, and even pet care.

QUICK CONTACT INFORMATION FOR PRACTITIONERS AND NUTRITION EDUCATION

Certified Nutrition Specialists from the American College of Nutrition

www.cert-nutrition.org
727-446-6086

American College for the Advancement in Medicine

www.acam.org
800-532-3688
714-583-7666

American Association of Naturopathic Physicians

www.naturopathic.org
703-610-9037
877-969-2267

American Academy of Environmental Medicine

www.aaem.org
316-684-5500

There are more than 5 million copies of Ann Louise Gittleman's books in print. She is one of the most prolific authors in the arena of health and healing with 25 books to her credit. She is an award winning author whose books *The Fat Flush Plan* and *Before the Change* appeared on *The New York Times* Bestseller's. She has appeared on "Dr. Phil," "The View," "20/20," "EXTRA," and "Good Morning America."

Index